D1330808

0 026 700 81X 28

Goodbye Mommy

Lora Lee Boynton

Goodbye Mommy

Memoirs of a Survivor

Matador
5 Weir Road
Kibworth Beauchamp
Leicester LE8 0LQ, UK
Tel: (+44) 116 279 2299
Email: books@troubador.co.uk
Web: www.troubador.co.uk/matador

ISBN 978-1848761-100

A Cataloguing-in-Publication (CIP) catalogue record for this book is available from the British Library.

Typeset in 11pt Book Antiqua by Troubador Publishing Ltd, Leicester, UK
Printed in Great Britain by the MPG Books Group, Bodmin and King's Lynn

Matador is an imprint of Troubador Publishing Ltd

ACKNOWLEDGMENTS

A heartfelt thank you to my parents and family who never gave up, to Peter for providing me a safe and loving environment to express myself, my sister Tina, Aunt Mimi, my dedicated medical team, and my lifelong friends for being there then and now.

A special thank you to author Helena Drysdale for making this book possible.

Autumn Light

I have swept the dead leaves
Of my gloomy grey days
Into the gutter
The refreshing autumn rains
Have washed them away.

In swaying silver branches
The sweet sugar song
Of an unseen bird
Echoes through cool sunny air,
A new and beautiful time.

In the coming days
Of chilling ice,
I will live in the snow-covered strength
Of the winter flower.

My once shallow roots
Have finally grown deep.
The firm hold of stubborn stability
Dares the weather of life
To challenge me now.

Lora Lee Boynton, November 1986 – Aged 16

Contents

Prologue

I could feel the cold slowly creep up the vein in my arm and when I could no longer feel its chill, I felt its poison weaken me; all the colour left my face, my temperature dropped and I began shivering uncontrollably. Suddenly weary, I shut my eyes while the toxins brought me to the edge of death.

'Oh God, I can't do this. I can't. Get me out of here. Please, I can't do it. I can't breathe. Make it stop,' I pleaded to Peter and no one in particular. Snot ran from my nose as I rocked and sobbed, rocked and sobbed.

My head was aching from the tight blue Cold Cap that was freezing my brain. Icicles formed on the protective gauze around my ears and forehead. I felt like I had a mouthful of ice that I couldn't spit out. The tightness of the cap, and the fact it was connected to a machine so I couldn't move about, made me claustrophobic. I clenched my fists as tightly as I could and scrunched my face, letting out a low growl of torment.

'It's not a choice, Lora Lee. You have to do this. You have to do this for our boys. For me. We need you. Come on darling, I'm here. Calm down. We'll do it together. Just breathe.' Peter stroked my leg.

He was right. I had to do this for my boys big and small. The prospect of not being there for my children consumed me with dread. It hurt to think of them growing up without me, a hurt more painful than the treatment I was enduring. So I changed my chant from, 'I can't do this' to 'You can do this Lora Lee. You can do it. Just concentrate on each breath. Rock and breathe. You promised your sons you would do whatever it takes. Do it for them. You know you can.' Somehow I managed to get through that difficult first hour.

It had been only a week and a half since the shocking diagnosis. Everything had proceeded at dizzying speed, and although I was desperately tired, the steroids I had been given to help with the induced nausea kept me awake. In an attempt to escape my surroundings, I sat in my uncomfortable cold vinyl seat with my eyes shut. I should have been able to extend the footrest so I could recline, but the room was too small. I went over events trying to make sense of the crushing deluge of grief. The smell of rubbing alcohol made my glands water and my stomach queasy. It catapulted me back to my youth and the pain I had been too young to name before.

I thought about the last time I suffered through chemotherapy 23 years ago when I was 15. Maybe it wouldn't have been so bad if Mommy had been there to reassure and hold me. I had felt so lonely. Every cell in my being ached for the protection of her, but Mommy was only a figment of my imagination.

My real mommy had abandoned my two sisters and me when I was only seven. This made me think about my own four sons and the possibility of abandoning them due to my illness. Telling my twelve-year-old the bad news was possibly the hardest thing I've ever had to do. He had just returned from a summer holiday with his father and my heart was full of dread as I heard his car pull up.

I had read pamphlets and websites on the best way to broach the subject with young children, but when it is your own child all that advice seems so weak and rehearsed. It was easier telling my three younger sons because they didn't really understand and didn't ask many questions, but my eldest has always been very sensitive, and I knew he would take it hard.

I recalled how I had thrown open our front door. 'Hi Darling. I missed you so much. How was your holiday?' I embraced him a little too eagerly and hugged him a little too hard. He didn't seem to notice; I was just being the overly doting mother he was used to.

'Yeah, it was good thank you. Dad made me walk everywhere. My legs are killing me.'

I flashed my eyes at his father James. I had already told him the news in a telephone conversation during their time away. James looked at me sadly. 'Here are PJ's things. His passport is in the bag. Alright son; hope you had a good time. See you in a couple of weeks.' James gave our son a hug, shot me another knowing glance, wished me well and left.

I shut the door slowly, reluctant to turn around and face PJ because tears were already welling in my eyes. I took a deep breath and tried to sigh away my sadness. We went into our living room and he sat in our large wingback chair while I kneeled on the floor beside him. We talked a little more about his holiday. He always came back so much more mature following time spent with his father. He appeared at least two inches taller and looked so grown up in his new jean jacket and gelled brown hair. His smooth baby-skin face was full of vibrancy and his unbroken voice reminded me that despite all his bravado, he was just a boy. While we talked I kept sucking in deep breaths and letting them out in huffs of agitation because I knew what had to be said.

'Is something the matter Mom?'

'Well, yes.' I said looking at him intently. I placed my hand on his knee and continued. 'Do you remember I told you I was having some tests done at the hospital?'

'Yeah, Dad said I shouldn't worry about it because lightening never strikes the same spot twice.'

That didn't make what I had to say any easier. I continued, 'I had the results back a couple of days ago.' I swallowed hard, feeling a huge lump in my throat, and widened my eyes urging him to fill in the gaps.

He looked away and stared at the floor. I let him collect his thoughts in silence and piece together what was coming next. He had recently witnessed my little sister's slow deterioration and endured the pain of losing her through illness, and now he was imagining losing me the same way. He began to shudder as tears streamed down his face.

When he could he said, 'I had a dream while we were in Germany. I could see you suffering behind thick glass but I couldn't break the glass to help you. I was forced to stand and watch you die.'

'Oh honey,' I said as I grabbed him in my arms. We held each other tightly both crying.

'Are you going to die like Aunty Cake did?'

That was the question I was dreading most. What do I say? I couldn't lie and tell him everything was going to be fine. What if it wasn't? What if despite all my reassurances, I ended up suffering and dying like my sister had? I answered by saying that I was going to do whatever it takes to be here for him and his brothers in the future. That we should just look at this period in our lives as a difficult blip that will pass.

'Mom, is there a chance you may die?' he asked again more forcefully.

Reluctantly I said, 'Yes, I suppose there is, but I swear to you sweetheart if I have anything to say about it I'll be fine. I'll do everything in my power to get myself better. Whatever treatment it takes, I'll have it. I promise.'

My shoulder was damp from tears. 'Oh darling, I'm so sorry. Please don't cry.' I held onto him tightly. 'This kind of cancer is much more treatable than the cancer I had when I was a young girl. Statistically I have a higher chance of beating breast cancer than I did Ewings Sarcoma, and I beat that didn't I?'

PJ told me he had a friend at school whose mother was diagnosed for the second time with breast cancer and the outcome looked bleak. I explained that this is the nature of breast cancer – it can come back at any point however long you've been in remission or cured.

'So it's not just a blip then, is it?' he asked in an accusing tone.

I didn't reply and PJ didn't say anything more. After twenty minutes or so I let go of him and wiped his tears with my hands. 'I love you, son. Please don't worry.'

'Do you mind if I go to my room to be alone for a while?'

'Of course not, but remember if you want to talk or ask any questions I'm right here.' As he left, I felt my shoulders slump and my head fall under the weight of my burdens. All my energy was depleted; even the thought of standing felt too daunting so I sat staring across the room. How could this be happening? Oh God, how did I get to this point? I pulled my knees up towards my chest and wrapped my arms around my legs. Fearing the worst, I heard my body let out an inhuman sound of agony.

I heard a nurse impatiently ask Peter to move out of the way again so she could get to the fridge that held all the drugs. I heard him say very politely, 'sorry.' It made me angry that he was apologising when I was a private patient having to go through treatment in such cramped surroundings.

I opened my eyes and saw poor Peter sitting there on a little stool in our tiny overheated room while I endured what I had to. He sat there for hours but he never once complained. I knew he had work he could have been getting on with, but on treatment days he put aside his own agenda and made it all about me. I can honestly say if it weren't for him sitting by me, supporting and soothing me, I would have ripped out every last tube and chosen to die.

'I've got to make a call to the office darling. Is there anything I can get you?' he asked sweetly.

'The ulcers in my mouth are really hurting. Can you get me some ice to suck on?'

'Sure,' he said kissing me softly on my forehead.

After he left, I sighed heavily. I pulled at the Cold Cap seeking even the slightest relief from the cold. I hated wearing it but knew it would delay any hair loss, so it had to be worth it. I felt agitated at having to be in such a filthy place full of illness, foul smells, and people from all walks of life. Even the outside garden was strangled with weeds and overgrowth. The small pond on the patio was stagnant; a perfect nesting ground for mosquitoes and a great way to spread disease. What made me most angry was that some of us were spending our very last precious moments in such negative and unhappy surroundings. Surely the NHS could do better than this! A huge part of recovery is feeling positive, but how does one feel positive sitting in a toilet bowl? I used to say to myself that I am as tough as old boots, and that is how I pulled myself through some trying times in life. The truth is, I could not bear the idea of being a victim. The word seems to imply that I have no control, no options left to me, no way out. I did have options: I could put up barriers and keep myself safe and protected within.

I was ashamed of where I had come from, never wanting to acknowledge my past. All the homes my two sisters and I lived in, the terrible situations we found ourselves in because my mother was a drunk, being abandoned for the last time when I was only seven, and being separated from my sisters: these were all memories I wanted to forget. I had been lost without my sisters – hadn't known what to do on my own or how to be Lora Lee without them. I was old enough to have vivid memories of being torn from them, but too young to articulate all the pain and hurt. I didn't even know what I was supposed or allowed to feel. Something in me had shrivelled up and died. I would never be the same again.

Without even realising it, I had disconnected myself from that abandoned little girl and pretended my life before adolescence was just a bad dream. I felt like I was looking down on myself through the wrong end of a pair of binoculars; I looked so small and distant. I wanted to believe I was normal -- needing to fit in and belong somewhere. I wanted to be accepted for who I was now – not who I was then (never connecting in my mind that it was the same person). The once clingy seven-year-old who retreated into her shell was the same clingy adult still hidden away. Becoming invisible, I mastered numbness and became almost unreachable to everybody, including me. If I could fool myself, I would be able to fool others. Just don't look too closely and all will seem normal. I was so lost, depressed, frightened of my own shadow, scared to live and downright stressed out and unhealthy, and I didn't even realise it.

Finding out for the second time in my life I had cancer blew the lid off my pressure cooker. I was only 36 and had many things to figure out, and I needed to do it fast because I might die. I didn't know how to stop the pain from coming and spilling over into everyday life. I kept thinking if the cancer wasn't going to kill me, all the pain would. I knew it was no use. I could no longer shrug off the notion that emotional trauma from my childhood was affecting my physical health. If I was going to survive cancer physically and emotionally, I had to embrace my past.

No longer content to let anybody else speak for me or remain silent in my personal hell, I needed an outlet for all the pain. Never very good at speaking, always too shy and insecure, I turned to writing. Writing became my engine to get me through. Slowly my splintered memories came out and my wounded heart began to heal. I found my voice, and my strengths started coming back to me.

This book is about the slow realisation that life is about the journey – not just surviving or arriving. It is about reconnecting with the wounded child inside, taking an emotional flat line, a desolate cell of a heart, and making it pound loudly again. It is a book about bridging the past with the present, a book about life and loving.

Chapter 1

Places

I see my life in terms of the places I have lived, which totals well over 20 before the age of seven. My mother, two older sisters and I moved every couple of months, either because Mom couldn't afford to pay rent, or because the house was condemned. Sometimes we moved to find her a new job, or to get away from some man she had befriended and turned out to be a creep. It wasn't just homes we moved from, it was entire States. My earliest faded memories from when I was just four are of Massachusetts, while my clearer memories from the next few years are of Santa Rosa, California, and at one point Alabama.

Our various residencies were more like places than homes, because that is all they were to me – a place of shelter and a place to sleep, a place usually not even heated. We never had any inviting niceties that make a house a home. If the place had carpets, Mom told us not to sit on them because they were so filthy, but often the floor was cold vinyl or even dirt. We were taught very young how to hover over a toilet bowl to do our business, making sure not to touch any part of our body to the toilet seat in case it might pass on some undesirable disease.

In Massachusetts around 1974, we lived in two-bedroom places –

one room for Mom and her current boyfriend, and one for my sisters and me. Because we were youngest, Sheila and I shared the bottom bunk, while Tina slept on top. At weekends and during school holidays, Mom would send all of us for a nap even though Tina was nine and Sheila six. We rarely did fall asleep; it was far too much fun bouncing on the beds and playing racing cars. With two of us lying on our backs, we put our feet together and pressed one foot hard against the other's to accelerate or break. Because I was always at the headboard end and was the smallest, I was the one who was always revved into a hard spot. As long as we were out of her way, it didn't matter to Mom that we were making so much noise and having fun. Not long after we came out of our room, we were usually told to go back and clean it, even if it was already spotless.

Once Mom shouted at us to clean up every last piece of dust. 'I don't want to see one thing when I come back!' she hollered. Sheila said she must have really meant it, so we took everything we owned and threw it out the window of our second story apartment. At age 5, I thought it was the right thing to do, but I am fairly certain Sheila and Tina knew exactly what they were doing. Whatever it was they were trying to achieve backfired, though. When Mom found out, we had to go and fetch everything and take it back to our room – which worked out well for Mom because it meant we were preoccupied and once again 'out of her hair,' as she used to say.

Even though it was early to mid 1970's, the décor inside the places we lived suggested it was possibly the late 50's and early 60's with vinyl seats and tables with chrome legs and coated Formica tops. The basic appliances we did own spoke of another era, one where radio was the prominent source of entertainment and cars were built to last. Everything was big, shiny, and heavy. The first song I learned to sing wasn't a lullaby; it was 'All Shook Up' by Elvis Presley. Mom still backcombed her jet-black dyed hair during a time when it was trendy to let it grow long and natural.

We had enough to get us by — basic food, electricity, clothes bought from the local second hand shop and most importantly, we had each other. That was enough even when most others would consider it wasn't. If we were lucky, we had a couch to sit on and a small black and white television propped up on an old beer crate. Mom always found old furniture she would renovate. When she had finished, she would show me her latest masterpiece.

'Look Tiger! Isn't it great?' she said to me one day.

I wasn't an expert, but said, 'Isn't it suppose to have a middle drawer?'

'Awe,' she said looking down to the ground half ashamed. 'I know, but I did the best I could. At least we have a place to put some of our clothes now.'

She was right, it was better than the cardboard boxes we had to use sometimes. I was thankful for that.

A couple of years later there were improvements in the décor, but a distinct lack of space in return. Most places were small trailers or studio apartments with a kitchen and a small bathroom that had only a hand basin and shower. In the one room that served as living room and bedroom to all four of us plus Mom's current boyfriend, there was a big bed for my sisters and me, and a couch for Mom.

Mom acquired and proudly displayed a lit lava lamp in the corner of the room; its red, orange, and yellow bubbles floating and descending lazily. I loved looking for new shapes; I felt content and calm – how I imagine a foetus would feel tumbling effortlessly in the warmth of its mother's womb.

The curtains were nearly always drawn and incense burned to hide the smell of the joints Mom smoked. Whilst playing her favourite Eagles song, Hotel California, Mom danced with me, singing the lyrics as she twirled me around. The warm glow from her lava lamp, and the smell of incense burning its magical floral fragrance, surrounded us in heavenly sweet warmth, creating an intimate just us feel. The long strings of colourful glass beads that hung between the main room and the kitchen jingled and tinkled, advertising Mom's or my sisters' presence. The atmosphere made me feel good inside, like warm spicy mulled wine. I was blissfully unaware that there was anything better. I was happy and Mom and my sisters were all that mattered. What I wouldn't give to be there just one moment longer. I had no idea what was really brewing.

Chapter 2

Earliest memory

My earliest clear memory dates back to when I was four, when we lived in a trailer with two bedrooms in Fitchburg, Massachusetts. It was summer time, and Mom couldn't afford childcare, so she regularly left Tina, just short of age nine, in charge of Sheila and me while she went to work all day.

It was a hot day, the kind so dry it makes your nostrils ache, and Mom told Tina she was NOT under any circumstances to take us to the lake. Translation to young ears: *The lake is a really neat place, but you can't go... this is a challenge!*

After being indoors for some time and suffering from the sweltering heat, Tina got us dressed and in no time we were making our way towards the lake. On the way, Tina made us promise to stick together and look after one another. We vowed never to tell Mom where we had been.

All I know is one moment I was standing in ankle deep water looking at a spot down the beach that was busy with splashing and laughing young swimmers thinking, *Oooh, that looks fun!* Then I was bobbing uncontrollably up and down in the water where I had just been looking. Every time I came up just above

5

the water's surface, where I could see the sky, land, and children, I thought, *I'm going to shout* but instead only managed to swallow lungs full of water. I could see hundreds of tiny bubbles rising before me as I quickly began going down in the olive-brown water. It actually felt rather peaceful. I stopped fighting and let my body sink further into the depths. I was thinking how I should have stayed where I was when everything went black. There was nothing. Everything ceased to exist – even me.

The next thing I recall, I was lying on the beach vomiting water while someone was pumping my stomach. As I slowly regained consciousness, I opened my eyes and the sun was shining so brightly behind this person that all I could see was a dark silhouette with a bright corona of shining light. I thought it was an angel, but as I fully came to I realised my angel was none other than Tina. She told me she suddenly had a sixth sense that I was in trouble and frantically looked for me. She saw my arms flailing in the water and managed to save me at the very last second.

True to my word, I never told Mom what had happened. It was our sisterly secret.

Around the same time, I climbed out of bed whilst the rest of the house slept. I wore a large white t-shirt of Mom's and pink underwear as I padded across the cold vinyl floor in my bare feet to some toys on the other side of our bedroom. I played on my own for some time when I decided I couldn't wait any longer: I needed food. Not wishing to disturb anybody, I went through the fridge and settled on a small frozen chicken pie. I removed its packaging and placed it on a paper plate – how Mom always served it to me. Against my better judgement (I knew there was something not quite right about what I was about to do), I placed the pie on the oven burner and turned on the gas. The plate caught fire. In a state of panic I quickly grabbed a tea towel to put out the flames. The towel ignited. I threw the towel and watched it land on the counter under the kitchen window, igniting the lace curtain. I thought, *Oh No, Mommy's going to kill me!* I was scared. 'MOMMEEEE!' Thank God, Mom was there in no time, controlling what could have been another near death situation.

My beautiful mother looked like Jacqueline Smith, the long brown-haired woman from the original *Charlie's Angels* TV show. To me she was as soft as a doe with carob brown eyes full of naïve warmth and vulnerability. I thought the world of her; nothing she did swayed me from the belief that she was the most amazing and beautiful woman in the world.

Unfortunately, nothing could have been further from the truth. She was a hard woman with a serious drink and drug problem, but she didn't know it; or at least, she didn't admit it. Mostly it was her day-to-day habitual drinking that really impaired her judgement, making her useless at her job as our mother. For instance, she regularly sent me, age four, to the market to buy her cigarettes because she was too busy drinking with friends to do it herself. I would take a note giving me permission to buy cigarettes on her behalf. Blissfully I bounced along to a beat in my mind reciting out loud the small list of other things she'd asked me to get: 'a stick of butter, loaf of bread, milk and a pack of Marbelows... a stick of butter, loaf of bread, milk and a pack of Marbelows.' I didn't know how to say Marlboroughs. It was a long walk; I definitely wouldn't forget the list by the time I got there.

I bought the things she had asked for, but because I was so nervous forgot to buy the butter. As I left, I realised I was so focussed on remembering the list, I hadn't paid attention to how I got there. *Which way is it out of here?* Frightened of making the wrong choice and getting lost, I decided to hang out at the market for a while. I eyed a packet of cherry cough drops that looked yummy, wandered around the fruit and vegetable department taking in all the beautiful colours and fruity scents, and roamed the isles amongst things I'd never seen before.

I was always easy going. I had already learned that if you give situations long enough things eventually sort themselves out, and in this case I was right. Mom appeared out of nowhere grabbing my arm angrily, nearly lifting me off the floor as she dragged me out the store. I didn't bother explaining, she wouldn't have listened anyway.

Chapter 3

My sisters

Tina had dark brown, shoulder length hair, a turned up nose, thick ruby red lips, and striking mid-blue eyes. Sheila and I looked nearly identical with stringy, shoulder length blond hair, turned up noses, thin lips, and pale blue eyes. Sheila had a slightly chunkier and shorter build than I, with noticeably chubby cheeks, so Mom called her 'Chip' short for Chipmunk. Although Sheila and I looked very similar, we couldn't have been more different in character. Sheila was a headstrong, confident bully, whereas I was shy and insecure, and as a result tended to giggle nervously.

My sisters and I wore an odd assortment of clothes bought from second hand shops. I liked to wear pastel vertically striped trousers with a horizontally striped top in primary colours. I had a perpetually runny nose that I wiped on the sleeve of my bright pink polyester coat with fake blond fur around the hood.

A tight pack and a formidable force amongst the other local children, my sisters and I loitered a lot. We were tough and governed by a lack of rules. Other children did not mess with any one of us without suffering serious consequences. Let me just say, we were the ones your mother always warned you about. We were so feared that other children parted crowd on the sidewalk to let us through as we sang in harmony Barry Manilow's song, 'Can't smile without you, can't laugh, and I can't sing, I'm finding it hard to do anything.' We always sang, whether we were washing dishes, or parting crowds. Other favourite songs were, 'Country Roads' by John Denver, 'Don't it Make My Brown Eyes Blue' by Crystal Gale, and 'Teddy Bear' and 'All shook up' by Elvis Presley. When we sang 'Teddy Bear' I would sing 'hot bananas' in a deep voice trying to mimic the back up vocalists.

One summer's day in Massachusetts, whilst Mom was styling my hair into her favourite Shirley Temple curls, Tina announced she was going to fight a girl down the street. We were all excited for her; even Mom told her to give us a good name. After Tina left, we ran to the tall Victorian windows at the front of our living room, pressing our left cheeks to the glass trying to catch a glimpse of the fight down the street. About twenty minutes later, Tina arrived back with two fists full of dirty-blond hair. Pumped full of adrenaline, she told us how the girl she had fought was so gross she had lice, 'See,' she said showing us the hair in her hands.

One snowy winter's day at our local park in Fitzburg, my sisters and I came across our cat that had been missing for some time. Run over and in pancake form, our cat was frozen into a black and white disk that somebody had leaned against a wheelie bin. We were frightfully matter of fact about it, showing a real lack of emotional response, which was strange considering it had been our family pet. We kicked it around a bit and watched it slide over the iced sidewalks pretending we were playing ice hockey. Even by this age we were emotionally numb, a technique we would perfect throughout our lives in order to survive.

Looking back, I realise there was no doubt about it. We were a singular unit – each one not functioning without the other. As a unit, we protected and supported each other. Simply put, we were best friends. We took lead from each other. If one was sad, we were all sad. If Mom punished one of us, we took the punishment together. In many ways, Mom was the outsider and we were the family.

Chapter 4

Another move, another place

Still in Massachusetts, it was 1975 and we had moved to yet another place — a large Victorian house divided into apartments. I was blissfully unaware that there was an entire world out there. My personal headlines read, 'We move yet again' and 'Lora Lee has a bed-wetting problem.' Each night I went to bed and spent at least an hour worrying, determined it wouldn't happen again. Of course it always did. Mom tried spanking me, then tried making me do chores like sweeping the wooden floors. She even bought me a new mattress hoping that would help. It didn't. I was insecure and disturbed. What I really needed was some stability in my life, but I didn't know that and certainly would not have known how to communicate it other than by wetting my bed at night.

My sisters and I had some fun at this place. On a hot summer's day, Mom half filled two new large green rubbish bins with cold water, and Sheila and I were placed in one bin and Tina into the other. The lids were on, and the sunshine shone through the sides of the bin illuminating us in a wash of moss green. I remember the happiness in my sisters' faces as we clung to each other while Mom's boyfriend rocked the rubbish bins. What could be more fun? Our shrieks and giggles could be heard for a block in any direction.

That winter my sisters and I went for a walk to the park to throw snowballs. Bundled from head to toe, I kept my head down and my chin tucked in to shield my face from the achingly cold wind. I watched my sisters' shadows but couldn't hear them well because the hood of my jacket was pulled over my earmuffs. Slowly I walked on pushing into the wind. After a while of shuffling through thick snow, I looked up and realised my sisters were nowhere to be seen, and I had no idea where I was. I stood on the corner of a street lined with maple trees laden in snow. I was cold, scared and didn't know what I should do, so I employed my usual tactic and just stood there hoping the situation would sort itself out. It did. A kind elderly woman came to me and asked me where my mommy was. I explained to her that I was lost, that my sisters had abandoned me. She took me by the hand and led me to her home.

Inside her warm and deliciously aromatic kitchen, she offered me some chocolate chip cookies and milk. This was the first time I had been in such a beautiful and welcoming home with carpets, plants, and heating. There was a soothing stillness, a sense of stability I had never known before. I contently sat on a stool, legs dangling, eating my cookies and chatting with this very nice woman. I never knew a home could be so luxurious and safe. If she didn't figure out where I lived, I wondered if I could live with her happily ever after.

After I finished eating my cookies, she asked me, 'Do you think you could lead me to your home?' I looked at her doubtfully. She added quickly, 'I promise I'll stay with you and hold your hand. You won't get lost again.' With this reassurance I agreed to try to find my way back to Mom.

It turned out home was only around the corner, but nothing was familiar because the snow had covered it up. When I arrived back home with a strange woman holding my hand, Mom acted as if it was a normal occurrence and laughed it off. I'll never forget how happy I felt sitting in the nice woman's kitchen. It remains a fond memory, giving me something to aspire to and recreate in my own home.

Chapter 5

Mom and me

I don't have many memories of being alone with Mom. Usually it was when she had dropped my sisters off at school and was driving me home, or my sisters were out playing and I had just awoken from a nap. One day in our apartment in Rhonert Park following my nap, Mom made me some Lipton tea with two spoonfuls of sugar and invited me to sit with her on our couch. She began chatting to me about life. I couldn't really make sense of what she was talking about, but I felt so privileged to be on the receiving end of this important conversation. Suddenly, as if things were going so well, she took a joint out of her wallet, lit it, and took in a couple of short breathy sucks. Whilst trying to hold the smoke in and not cough, she handed me the joint, urging me to take it. I was nervous, knowing it was wrong, but I didn't want to spoil the moment and let Mom down. I certainly didn't want her to think I was chicken, so I took it, copied what she had done and handed it back.

I had four hits off her joint before everything started going fuzzy. I couldn't stop giggling at the confusion of sights, sounds and emotions I was experiencing. I felt like an electrical toy whose circuit was malfunctioning. The sound of her voice became a distant echo, and the lightening flashes in my retinas sent me into an emotionally frantic goose chase trying to understand what was happening to me. In the end, desperate to gain some control over my body, I laid down on the couch. As if in prayer, I tucked my hands under my head, shut my eyes and listened to Mom laugh. Eventually she left me and even though I had just awoken from a nap, I fell to sleep.

One memory with Mom sticks out above all others. Mom drove us along a bumpy dirt track on the edge of a cornfield. I sat next to her on the white vinyl bench seat of her 1950's baby blue Ford, my hair flapping in the wind. I could see Mom was experiencing a sense of freedom by the speed we were driving and the huge smile on her face.

'Hey – want to see how an old grandma drives?' she asked mischievously.

I bobbed my head up and down. I rarely saw Mom so playful and I was excited by what she might do next. I could tell by the glint in her eye that this was going to be fun.

She hunched over, put a false grimace on her face, stepped on the accelerator and waggled the steering wheel. The fringe on her leather jacket swayed as the car lurched from side to side. Great plumes of dust billowed up and I felt like we were starring in a TV episode of The Dukes of Hazard. I looked at her and thought *she's Elvis, Steely Dan and the Eagles. My mom's rock and roll!*

Unfortunately, the police officer watching from his patrol car hidden behind some shrubs didn't think she was so hot; at least, not until he pulled us over and started chatting with her. Mom explained what she was doing, smiled sweetly, played with her long dark hair, blinked her pretty carob droplet eyes in his direction, and he said, 'OK maam. Just remember you have a child with you.' Mom promised she would be more careful in the future and drove off in capable mother mode. Once the police officer was out of sight she looked at me and winked. They always fell for her act. Always.

We drove a bit further before Mom parked. 'Hop out Tiger — we're goin' fishing.' As we made our way to an elusive fishing spot, Mom explained that by entering from the east side of the bridge we couldn't possibly have seen the large 'No Fishing' sign facing the other direction. This was our story and we were sticking to it. We walked half way across the humpback wooden bridge and dropped our gear. After Mom hooked the worms, she cast a line for herself and then for me. We sat with our legs dangling over the edge of the bridge. Feeling no need to speak, we listened to the water rush downstream, and the cheerful songs of the birds in the surrounding trees. It was a warm and peaceful day — not too hot, not too cold. My eyes followed pieces of cottonseed as they churned effortlessly on a whisper of a breeze and landed lazily on the water. For once I knew where I was; I was safe and at peace sitting next to my mom.

Out of the blue I had a tug on my fishing line that nearly pulled me off the bridge. Mom jumped to her feet in wild excitement, taking over pole duty. I watched the pole nearly bend in half then suddenly the fish flew out of the water, snapping the pole back in the opposite direction. A gargantuan fish, bigger than me, sailed over our heads in what seemed to be slow motion, finally snapping the pole in two. Pulled by inertia and gravity, the fish and broken pole flew into the waters behind us on the other side of the bridge. It all happened in a matter of seconds as we stood there looking at each other with exhilaration in our eyes, 'Oh my God, did you see that Mom? Did you? It was huge!'

'Woo – hoo! That was a big 'un — high five!' she said holding her hand up. I smacked it and she said, 'Rock on!'

Too excited to fish, we packed up our things, one fishing pole lighter, and talked about the fish the whole way home. Each time she told the tale of the fish, the fish got larger. Soon it was as big as a shark, but I didn't say anything because it was more exciting that way.

Chapter 6

Uncle Dick

Shortly after our fishing trip Mom dropped me off at her brother Dick's house. I thought I was just staying the weekend, but the weekend became weeks and weeks became months. I didn't understand. Did I do something to make her mad at me? Was I a bad girl? It turns out Tina was left with the person Mom bred her dog with, and I'm not sure where Sheila was left. This was the first of many times Mom disappeared for long periods; slowly it became normal.

Uncle Dick and Aunt Cindy had very few parenting techniques. One day I sauntered into their kitchen looking for a snack. I found some Cheese-it biscuits in a bowl on the counter, took a handful and began to eat them one by one. Uncle Dick suddenly appeared and shouted at me, 'What the hell do you think you're doing?' I told him I was eating some Cheese-its, and wondered how this could be wrong. He stormed out of the room and returned a minute later with a flexible willow tree branch and said, 'This will teach you a lesson. Turn around and touch your toes.'

I could feel my dress pull up my legs as I bent over, worried that my pants underneath were showing as I touched my toes.

Suddenly a searing pain tore across the back of my bare legs. Not once but three times I felt the switch tear at my skin.

He stopped and waited for me to cry, but to my own detriment I refused to give him the satisfaction that he was hurting me. When he realised he hadn't broken me he said, 'Maybe this will teach you not to touch things that aren't yours,' and switched my legs three more times. My lips hardened. Even at the tender age of five, I recognised the evil power Uncle Dick was trying to derive out of hitting me. In order to escape my distress and hatred towards him, I went to a place deep inside and managed to conceal my pain and hostility.

Uncle Dick switched me six more times when I began to feel something warm trickle down my legs. I was worried that perhaps I had wet myself, but to my horror I saw it was blood. Uncle Dick must have realised that he had crossed the line between sanity and madness because he stopped, but this wasn't the end of my punishment. He then made me open and shut a kitchen drawer for over an hour leaving my knuckles blistered, and finished with a lecture about not telling anybody what he had done.

It was impossible to hide my scabby legs whilst wearing my school uniform dress. When the Principal of my school promised nothing bad would happen if I explained to him how the scabs occurred on my legs, I reluctantly told him. When I arrived home from school that day, everything personal I owned – besides the clothes on my back – had been taken away. For a week they made me sit on my own in a barren room and sleep on a bed with no sheets and covers. I fell asleep in my school clothes night after night crying for the protection of my mommy, believing she would never have allowed them to hurt me like this. Even though she had left me, she must still surely love me. Didn't she?

Uncle Dick and Aunt Cindy's good parenting techniques didn't end there. My uncle lived on a large plot of land surrounded by forest on the northeast side and never ending fields on the other. They had a tyre swing hanging from a tree just outside their house that should have been fun but I dreaded it. Despite the fact it was the middle of winter, Uncle Dick told me on several occasions to sit on the tyre swing and not move until given permission. Although my bare hands were frozen blue and I desperately needed a toilet, I sat there alone for hours too frightened to move in case Uncle Dick switched me. Shivering and lonely in the pale blue evening light, I watched their house glow and wondered what was going on inside. Wishing I could be part of the warmth emanating through their windows, I thought I must be a really terrible person for them to hate me so much. I vowed that I would try harder to be the way they wanted me: invisible.

Their children weren't much better. They took me into the forest one day and convinced me there was a bear coming and left me there alone. Hidden amongst the trees, they made growling noises that terrified me. They crunched dry sticks and leaves under their feet making it sound as if a bear was close by and I panicked. I ran like the wind frantically trying to get away from the bear that was just out of sight. I was so engrossed in trying to get away that I didn't notice the board with a rusty nail sticking up out of it. I felt the nail pierce through my sneakers and go straight through my foot, but my surge of adrenaline masked the throbbing pain. Once back to the safety of Uncle Dick's house, I was shouted to get out of the house with my bloody foot. Aunt Cindy angrily removed my shoe to inspect my wound and said, 'there are no bears here you stupid child.'

It wasn't always so bad there, though. I was learning to concentrate on the upside of life. There were actually some fun things to do too. Once my cousins and I dug a deep trench trying to create a place where there was no sound. A couple of us got in, placed a board over the top and sat as silently as we could. We discovered that the quieter we tried to be, the louder the silence became.

We also enjoyed building go-carts out of Uncle Dick's collection of junk. I only remember one cousin well – David. I played with David most because he was closest in age to me. In particular we liked playing cowboys and indians. He was also the first boy to show me his willy. No, I didn't ask him to, but he thought I might be interested. I was, for about five seconds, and then decided the game we were playing was much more interesting.

It was whilst living with Uncle Dick that I started school for the first time. I could see the school building from his house far across the fields of swaying silvery brown in summer, and pea green grass during spring and autumn. In winter the school stood out magnificently amongst the spare white background of snow covered fields.

My first school day was pale yellow in early autumn and the maple leaves were beginning to turn and fall in the fresh breeze. The school was a large brick building with turning crimson ivy stretching its tentacles up the sides. Having found my classroom and taken my seat, a nice young blond woman asked me to come to her desk so she could ask me some questions. I happily bounced over believing school was fun and listened as she told me a little about herself, making me feel more comfortable. She then asked me a few questions like my name and age, which was easy, but when she asked me to identify the shape she was holding up, I stared at her blankly thinking, *Shape? What's a shape?*

'Is it a triangle or square?'

I took a stab, 'Triangle.' I now know it was a square.

She held up another shape and then another asking similar questions of me. I sensed by the way her blond eyebrows were increasingly stitching together that she had cottoned onto my little secret.

Later that day, she asked her students, including me sitting in the middle of the class eager and willing to learn, 'Does anybody have a song they would like to share with the class?' A few children stood up and sang, and I thought it was wonderful — I had never heard children's songs before and wanted to stand up and sing too. I raised my hand, and the teacher invited me to share my song. Brushing my stringy blond hair away from my eyes, I looked around at my fellow classmates, brought my hands together in front of me fidgeting my fingers nervously as I took a deep breath in and began my song, 'Once there was a teddy bear.'

The whole class sang, 'Once there was a teddy bear,' and waited for the next verse.

'Um, it's my teddy bear not my sister's,' I sang with less conviction.

The whole class repeated 'Um, it's my teddy bear not my sister's.'

'Ummmm,' I looked up into my head then looked down and fidgeted my fingers some more whilst waiting for lyrics to pop into my mind.

'I think maybe you have forgotten the words,' the nice blond woman said.

'Yes, I have' I said shyly not looking at her but at the floor instead. She extended an invitation for me to practice the song further at home and share it with the class later. I sat down feeling quite happy that I had contributed, and she even wanted me to sing it again!

Most of the time I played alone at Uncle Dick's house. I didn't mind; I enjoyed the quiet and found creative things to keep me busy. I took great pleasure in creating miniature cities using the clear plastic lids off the fruit Aunt Cindy bought, filling them with dirt and things I could readily find. I made little houses out of matchbooks, and pebble roads lined with maple trees. I used a lid from my coke bottle to create a small pool for the imaginary children to play in, and a small metal toy car to put in the drive of the home. On the house, I drew windows and curtains, and put grass in the front and back gardens. I finished it with some small flowers on either side of the front door. 'This is what a home should look like,' I whispered to myself as I moved the car around the pebble road.

Chapter 7

Reunited

The following September, still in Massachusetts, Mom, my sisters and I were reunited. One moment I had been living with Uncle Dick, and then without warning I was back with my family again as if nothing had ever happened. There was no discussion on why she left or how we were whilst she was away. She never even asked if we had enjoyed ourselves, or if we were happy, and it never occurred to me to share with her my experience. She was back, my sisters and I were together again, and that was all that mattered.

At first we lived in a simple trailer. I was hungry, but the only food I could find was dry dog food, so I shut myself in the pantry where it was kept and began to eat kibble by kibble. Mom caught me and thought it was hilarious. So hilarious, she demanded I get down on my hands and knees and act like a dog. I thought it was funny too, so I went along even giving a bark to authenticate my performance.

Not long after we moved to California. On an unforgettable summer's day during 1976, Mom took Sheila and me deep into the Redwoods to an area only hippies could love and showed us an incredible house. It wasn't a trailer or an apartment, but a proper house with lots of land surrounding it. Sheila and I inspected the empty rooms very carefully before coming up with a dream plan of where we would sleep, what we would play, and whom we would meet. As we looked around, we couldn't believe our luck when we discovered the windows had shades, and at the bottom of the shades were wooden sticks that slipped out from either end making useful weapons with which to slay each other.

Mom came into the room that would be our bedroom and asked us if we would be happy there. 'Yes!' we both squealed in delight, jumping up and down.

'If you are good girls, this will soon be yours!'

In the meantime, we were by now living on the Russian River sleeping in sleeping bags and catching our dinner fresh from the river. I fished for crawdads in the shallow waters, holding a fishing line with cheese as bait over the rocks. Too tempted to resist, a crawdad would come out very cautiously and as it tentatively pinched the cheese with one of its large front claws, I yanked hard pulling it out of the water. I loved catching them, but I couldn't bear watching Mom place them live into a boiling pot of water. Mom loved fishing and would spend the entire day catching catfish. Once she cut the belly open on one and hundreds of eggs poured out onto the cutting board. I was beginning to realise Mom must be a hard woman to be able to do something like that without even flinching.

Chapter 8

George

We were good girls, but instead of moving into the house we were promised, Sheila and I were flown to Alabama to live with our biological father, George, his wife Helen, and their children. Tina stayed with Mom because she had a different father than we did. On the plane, Sheila and I sat next to each other for the first hour or so. I could see the blinking lights on the end of the plane's wing, and commented to Sheila that we were obviously still on the ground. She replied, 'No were not. We're flying.' This started a monumental argument between us, one that resulted in hair pulling and the flight attendant separating us for the duration of the flight.

It was very early in the morning when George collected us from the airport. As we drove along the calm highway with lush green banks, I noted how different it looked to the busy heavily advertised highways of California. It was awkward being in a strange man's car not knowing where we were and what was expected. He kept talking and asking questions, but I ignored him and continued to stare out the window. Sheila nudged me with her elbow trying to get me to say something, but I was too engrossed in all the noise in my mind to pay attention. I kept wondering when I was going to see Mom again; I already missed her and felt hollow inside. I began to suck my thumb for comfort, even though I knew that would have made Mom cross with me. I sucked my thumb so hard and often it changed shape from all the calluses. Mom used to take it out of my mouth at night and cover it in Tabasco sauce hoping that would deter me. In actual fact, all it did was make me crave spicy food. Even to this day, everything I eat is smothered in hot chilli sauce.

It was Christmas time, and for the first time in my life I saw and experienced Christmas in all its glory. I lay under the colourful baubles hanging from the bottom branches of the tree looking at my distorted reflection as the colourful lights blinked. Up until this point, the closest I had ever been to experiencing Christmas was the time in Fitzburg, Massachusetts when my sisters and I wrapped up all of our own toys and placed them around the base of some long wheat grass we had picked and put in a container. In particular, Tina had wrapped her electric organ and then unwrapped it the night before Christmas so we could sing *Silent Night* while she played. Thinking of this as the lights blinked on George's tree, I thought, *Wow! What else have I been missing out on?*

George was an Army Officer so we lived on an army base. It felt more like a miniature communist city: suppressed, controlled, devoid of colour, expression and class. Sheila and I regularly raided a central supply storeroom packed with camouflage green cans of food. We couldn't read, and there were no pictures on the tins, but we reorganised the storeroom to our liking, so we could find what we wanted if the need should ever arise. Accustomed to worrying about where the next meal would come from, this was a perfect solution.

It was at this place I started to believe school wasn't fun anymore and subsequently perfected the art of pretending to be sick. One day, in an effort to get out of going to school, I put my forehead over an open burner to warm my head. I accidentally burnt my fringe and in an effort to cover up my botched attempt at being ill, I took baby oil and poured it over my head. Thinking nothing more of it, I caught the morning yellow school bus. Within an hour of being at school the Principal called me into his office and asked me to explain why I had a greasy head, then sent me home to rectify the problem. It was at this point I adopted a new tactic: in the future I would use the heat from a light bulb to warm the thermometer.

In the evenings, a mix of maybe 9 or 10 local children, Sheila, our step siblings and I –would sit on the ground on the edge of a forest listening to Rod Stewart's song, *Tonight's the Night*. We thought the lyrics were quite naughty which made listening to it more fun. We also liked to sit on skateboards and barrel down some of the steeper roads without any means of stopping or controlling where we ended up. Many bruises were worn proudly as a statement of how tough we were. We were simply lucky a car hadn't hit us, or that we hadn't broken our necks.

It was during this time that Sheila became increasingly aware of boys. She showed me a magazine hidden under her mattress with an article about breasts. She explained that it said if we massaged our chests over and over we would grow big breasts. I wasn't sure if she made that up, but just in case I spent a lot of time in the future rubbing my chest. Just for the record, I did not at this point grown big breasts as a result.

George and my stepmother Helen drank too much and discussions quite often ignited into soaring heights of emotional despair. One night without any warning, Helen flew across the room screaming and crying, attacking George with all her strength, pounding her fists on his chest and shaking her head wildly from side to side. It all happened so fast that we, the children, didn't have time to leave the room. We watched in stunned silence. It ended with him grabbing her by the wrists, wrapping her arms around her waist, and holding her until she calmed down. Once he felt she was calm enough, he let her go and she slumped to the floor in defeat, head hanging low, crying quietly. He kneeled in front of her and lifted her head with his forefinger so she was looking into his eyes. He spoke in a masculine hushed tone, brushing her wet snotty hair away from her eyes while we snuck out quietly to our rooms and lay on our beds trying to digest what we kept witnessing.

I believe it was the break up of George and Helen's marriage that forced Sheila and me back with Mom in California. This time the plane wasn't the large commercial airliner we flew to Alabama in, but a small four-seat private jet. Sitting behind the pilot, we bumped along through the night flying just above the clouds. I could see the lights on the end of the plane's wings and realised Sheila was right after all. Soon after take off she and I were once again bickering and the pilot had to shout for us to settle down or we were going to crash. We didn't say one word after that.

When we arrived at San Francisco Airport, Mom ran up and greeted us with great big bear hugs. I wrapped my arms around Mom's neck and breathed in her sweet vanilla scent feeling a huge sense of relief wash over me. I was so happy to hold my mommy and feel her warmth again. Unfortunately her mood quickly changed when she smelled the cheap cologne whose bottle had broken in Sheila's bag. 'What is that shit?' she asked opening Sheila's wet bag. 'Right. In the bin; all of it.'

'No Mommy, please!' I begged her as she began putting all our new toys in the bin. My plea teetered on desperation as I grabbed her arms to save my Barbie doll.

'You can keep the Barbie but the rest goes. Same for you Sheila,' she said throwing away all the other toys indiscriminately as we stood and watched.

I couldn't understand why it was necessary to throw the toys out. She touched them as if she was holding a hot potato and she couldn't get rid of them fast enough. I thought she would be happy we had some toys to play with, but her reaction told me she either resented the reminder of what she couldn't offer us, or the image of the man that gave them to us. Either way, she couldn't bear the emotions the toys were causing her so they had to go.

Not long after that, I cut the hair off my Barbie, and when I realised her hair wouldn't grow back, I hid her under our mattress and stole Sheila's doll saying it was mine. When Sheila discovered what I had done, she never let me forget my dishonesty. Indeed to this day she still brings up 'the hairless Barbie.'

Chapter 9

The year I would never forget

It was early 1977 when Sheila and I returned from George's and were reunited with Mom and Tina in California. We proceeded to live in four different places, the nicest being a two-bedroom apartment in a newly-built complex in Rohnert Park near Santa Rosa. Mom shared her bedroom with her boyfriend while my sisters and I shared a bedroom. I remember running my hand through the beige fibres of the new carpet, appreciating how clean it was. We even had a separate kitchen/dining and living room. I don't know how Mom could afford such a decent place on a bartender's salary; she must have been supplementing her income another way.

My sisters and I spent entire days in the surrounding fields making huge bird nests out of the long brown wheatgrass. The smell of fresh grass, mixed with warm sunshine and internal peace reminds me of a wholesome breakfast cereal advert. On other days, we walked across the field to a Hippy community to help in the health food store. By filling bags full of pulses, grains, and nuts we earned 25 cents each. The manager was a middle-aged, longhaired man, who had one normal arm and one tiny useless arm, but we didn't make much of it at the time.

Furthermore, I don't recall making much of the fact that everybody, including him, walked around naked. I guess seeing Mom's many boyfriends walk around in the nude had hardened us to it.

With the money we earned, we went to the local 7 / 11 convenience store, bought 'Red Hots' candy, and pretended they were drugs that gave us energy. We mimicked what we had seen displayed by Mom or one of her many men by popping two into our mouths and throwing our head back like we were trying to swallow them. Sometimes we wouldn't bother working for money, we would just steal the candy. If Mom suspected we had stolen, she asked us to stick out our tongue, telling us she could tell if we were lying because white spots would appear. We believed her, so we always told her the truth, but oddly she never disciplined us for stealing so I don't know why she even bothered asking.

Also across the field was an abandoned, dilapidated barn Sheila and I liked to go to in search of treasures. It was an eerie chicken graveyard with hundreds of bones lying around, and nests full of un-hatched eggs. It appeared as if a farmer had just shut the door on a barn full of healthy chickens leaving them to die. We tried on several occasions to hatch the eggs, wanting something good to come from the situation, but when nothing happened we reluctantly took them to a ditch and threw them in. Bad mistake. I can smell their pungent, sulphuric odour even now.

One day Sheila and I hesitantly tip toed into the half lit crumbling building. The dark shadows and cobwebs made it look like a scene out of Arachnophobia where I knew a huge spider was cleverly biding her time before she would strike. We heard a low distant moaning and I clung to Sheila's arm as she insisted we move closer. 'I don't want to. I'm scared.' Something moved at my feet. I was trying to be brave like Sheila, but felt the panic

bursting in me and squealed to let it free. 'It's OK Lora Lee. I'm
here,' Sheila whispered. The door we had entered through
suddenly slammed behind us and I clung to Sheila as if my life
depended on it. Sheila said, 'There it is again. There's that sound.'
As I strained to hear, I thought I saw something move in a
shadowy corner. That was it. I turned and ran for the door leaving
Sheila behind.

Back outside in the sunshine and feeling more confident, I saw
Tina and her friends throwing pebbles into the barn through
cracks in the wall. They peered in through a gap and were trying
not to explode with laughter, doubling over holding their
stomach, as one of them would create a guttural sound. I
watched and giggled at a distance and when Tina saw me, she
came to me and acted as if she was stealing my nose between
her two fingers, 'You alright, squirt?' I nodded but was secretly
disappointed because I preferred the barn to be haunted.

Around this time, Tina started smoking and felt I should too. I
was only seven years old when I sat behind a metal stairwell and
Tina showed me how to hold a cigarette. I took the cigarette
from her between my middle and forefinger. I brought it to my
lips in the most grown up way I could, sucked in smoke through
my tight lips as if I was eating hot soup, swallowed and held my
breath before blowing it out again. Within seconds my head felt
faint and I became violently ill. I ran upstairs to our apartment,
threw open the front door and bolted to the loo where I threw
up. In between heaves I blurted out, 'Tina made me smoke!'
which got Tina into serious trouble.

To get out of Mom's way in the evenings, my sisters and I met the
other local children at the pool in our apartment grounds. We
sat next to the water, lit a bright blue at night, playing *Truth or
Dare* and *Spin the Bottle*. Because I was the naïve one, quite often
I was naked at the end of a game of *Spin the Bottle*, while

everybody else was still fully clothed. While we played our games, Mom was sat at our dining room table drinking and playing poker with friends. On the wall behind them hung a fold out from Playgirl of *Long Dong Silver.*

In the morning, I sat quietly eating my Rice Krispies examining *Long Dong's* dong, thinking how incredibly ugly it was. As I contemplated what Mom saw in men, I was vaguely aware of the lingering smell and taste of stale beer and cigarettes in the air. At least the house was tidy; the house was always tidy. Mom was very fastidious, probably because her father had been in the army. Whatever the reason, I finally inherited a good trait from her. To be fair, when she chose to be she was also an artistic soul who loved to sing and dance. I am a bit like that too, except I make an effort to be like that most of the time whereas she infrequently did.

I discovered around the age of seven I had an accurate sixth sense about things. Maybe it was because I was getting older and wiser, but I began to be able to predict what a person was going to do or say, or how a situation would pan out on its current course. I had this ability to feel what was really going on in any given situation; an ability and radar of mine that I learned very successfully early in life to dodge and ignore at all cost when it didn't tell me what I wanted to hear. Mom teased me for my sensitivities, telling me I was a sissy or chicken when I decided not to do something in fear of my inner voice. Although a shy girl, I knew and remained true to my own common sense even when Mom pressured me to sway. I believe she secretly respected me in that way because there were times when she too took heed from what I feared was going to happen.

Chapter 10

Distaste in men

One evening still at the same place, Mom made my sisters and me do a strip tease dance for her and her boyfriend. The main overhead bulb was replaced by a black-light that made everything glow purple, and a large glitter ball turned and sparkled causing an Alice in Wonderland effect. As the music played, my sisters and I giggled whilst we removed our clothes one piece at a time and threw them across the room. Mom and her boyfriend sat on the couch and watched. Mom thought we were funny and laughed, but the look on her boyfriend's face was more than just amused. In the end, my sisters and I were naked, wriggling to the beat of the music, showing off our clever dance moves.

I wasn't old enough to realise anything sinister was occurring, but I did raise an inward eyebrow when Mom's boyfriend asked Tina to sit on his own naked lap. As Tina did, happily wrapping her arm around his neck, I saw Mom's boyfriend put his hand high up between Tina's legs. Mom turned a blind eye and nobody else seemed to mind, so I dismissed what I had seen as something acceptable and normal.

A few nights later whilst Mom was out, the same boyfriend told

Tina to take her clothes off and lay naked with him on the floor in the living room. Tina was accustomed to being forced to do sexual favours for Mom's boyfriends. On this occasion, he didn't try to penetrate her, but pressed and rubbed his hard naked front against the small of her back as they lay in a spoon position. Tina tried telling Mom what he had done, but Mom became irate in disbelief. Telling her what horrible children we were, Mom tore up all of our photographs and forced Tina to take them to the large dumpster outside. Then she made Tina stay awake all night by continually splashing her in the face with ice water. Finally at 5:00 AM, when Mom realised her boyfriend wasn't coming home that evening and couldn't say Tina was lying, she gave up and let Tina sleep for an hour before we all had to get up and go to school.

The following day at school, Tina told one of Mom's friends what had happened and that Mom hadn't believed her. When we all returned home from school, Mom, her boyfriend, social services and the police were all present in our apartment. Mom's boyfriend was crying, and Tina shrunk in shame believing it was her fault that he was so upset. She felt she shouldn't have said anything because she was causing our family so much distress. She needn't have worried because Mom somehow twisted the story around. She told social services and the police that it was Tina who was mentally disturbed and not her boyfriend who had done something wrong. The government officials removed Tina from our home and placed her in care where she would remain for almost a year before being allowed to live with us again.

I could never understand why Mom hated Tina so much. It makes me ache for my dear sister who was only a little girl looking for love and safety from her mother. Emotionally abused by Mom, and physically abused by many of Mom's men, Tina never felt loved or wanted for one moment. Mom was cruel when she looked at Tina; her expression suggesting Tina didn't exist. When

Mom wasn't looking straight through or past her, it was a look of disgust, as if Tina was dirty.

Mom blamed Tina for all of her problems, and I blamed the men Mom dated for all of Tina's and hers. Men had become an annoying part of Mom that we learned to cope with. For me, men were weak, lacked morals and character, and were ruled by the head on their penis instead of the head on their shoulders. I never trusted any of them, even when they went to great efforts to get on my good side. The way they laughed, like how I imagine a weasel would look and sound if it could laugh, made my skin crawl. Tina says I should be thankful that Mom's men liked me so much; it is for that very reason Mom showed an interest in me too.

Once, sitting in Mom's pick up truck outside a store, her boyfriend asked me very politely if he could kiss my mommy. Embarrassed, I nodded yes. I expected him to kiss her softly and gently, maybe even pet her on her cheek with the back of his hand. Instead, he proceeded to try and eat her face, sticking his thick tongue aggressively down her throat, groping her breast with one hand while I sat next to them and watched. I rolled my eyes up to heaven and breathed a heavy sigh wishing somebody or something would take away the feeling of distaste flooding my soul.

On another day, Mom and I stood with some of her friends on the porch of a Victorian house in which we were renting a room. They were talking about favourite colours. Mom's boyfriend, who had long brown hair, rotten front teeth and wore cut off jean shorts and no top, looked at me as he sat on a porch swing. He spoke through his nose, sniggering, 'This is my favourite colour,' moving his shorts to the side exposing his naked manhood. He seemed so proud of himself, whereas I felt complete revulsion, wrapping my arms around Mom's legs and hiding my face so he couldn't see how much I disliked him. Believing I was just being shy, Mom and the rest of her friends laughed.

There was a short time, too, when Mom disappeared altogether and my sisters and I were living with a strange man and his mother. By this point I was emotionally numb and disconnected inside. I had long stopped questioning why Mom was gone or who we were with now or why. It had become the norm to wake up in different places each day and have no routine. In order to cope, I stopped caring about anything. The end result was that I didn't know how I felt, didn't know who to cling to when I was upset and lonely. I was insecure, defenceless, exposed, and frightened – especially of the strange man we were living with now. I cannot help think there are memories about this man that I have blocked out entirely because for years I had bad dreams that he was coming to get me and I don't know why. I ask myself repeatedly what made me so petrified of him, but no answers come.

For a long time I thought the memories I harboured of being rescued from a strange man's house were just another one of my bad dreams; that it hadn't really happened. But I remember it all clearly now. I can see the lightening and the horizontal downpour of rain. I can feel the rumble of the thunder and the cold of the room. It was the middle of the night when I felt Mom shake me.

'Shhhh' she said holding her finger to her lips. 'Don't make a sound.'

I looked at Mom through sleepy, blurry eyes believing I was having a wonderful dream that my mommy had come to rescue me.

'Mommy?'

Mom said nothing, taking a blanket and wrapping it around me and putting my shoes quickly onto my feet. Before I knew it, we were outside in the pouring rain heading down a muddy hill between shrubs and through thick undergrowth. Thunder rumbled and lightening flashed, forcing my heart into my throat.

Mom kept talking about someone following us, that 'he' was coming for us and 'he' wanted to hurt us. With eminent danger nipping at my heels, I held Mom's hand and moved as fast as my little legs would carry me. At the bottom of the hill, my sisters and I were bundled into a waiting car and taken to my aunt's trailer. Mom told us not to turn on any lights or make a sound. As my sisters and I laid on a pull out bed, I shook from the rush of adrenaline and fear. I was willing my heart to stop pounding so loudly in case it might be heard when I heard Mom say, 'Shit, he's cut the phone line.'

I don't ever remember feeling that frightened again, not even today.

Up until the point of being dramatically rescued, we had been living with this man whose name none of us can remember. We remain unclear as to how or why we ended up with him. Tina says Mom gave us to him, and judging by an email that Mom sent me much later in life, I believe she may not be far off. In fact, I think it is even worse than that. I believe she accepted $10,000 from this man in return for us. She sold us, saying it was something to do with being accepted back into the Catholic Church, but more importantly, she seemed to want to get away from another mystery man and needed the money to do it.

Having been dramatically stolen back from the nameless man, Mom, Sheila, and I lived in a single bedroom apartment above a disco in downtown Santa Rosa. Tina was once again living somewhere else so it was just Sheila and me sharing a tiny bedroom while Mom slept on a couch in the kitchen/lounge. Some nights after I showered, I would go to say goodnight to Mom, but she was already having sex with her current man. The visions I try to forget of Mom kneeling with her bare bottom pointed at me whilst she performed oral sex have haunted me my entire life. My distaste for men quadrupled that precise moment because I was certain that Mom wasn't to blame for not saying goodnight to me. Men always took my beautiful mommy away. She was only a victim of their perverse demands. I mean, couldn't he even wait long enough for me to get in bed? Didn't he know she had children?

Mom did have one boyfriend I was fond of. Jerry. The only boyfriend whose name I can recall. He was kind to me in an, *I'm such a cool hardcore biker dude with long hair* kind of way.

Jerry had just returned from a liquor store in Santa Rosa, having stolen a bottle of 7 Crown whiskey. Listening to Steely Dan in our small apartment laden in cigarette smoke, Mom, Jerry and a couple of others finished the 7 Crown in no time. One man was heavily frothing at the mouth, and I asked Mom what was wrong with him. She said it was because he was allergic to alcohol and shouldn't be drinking. It was distressing to watch them continue to fill his glass despite the obvious threat to his life. I couldn't understand it. In fact, there were many things happening around me that I didn't understand and was beginning to question.

After the 7 Crown was finished, Jerry was leaving to go steal another. I had a strong premonition and begged him not to go, hanging onto his legs as long as I could. Following loads of laughter from the peanut gallery, he shook me off his leg and went to the liquor store. Sure enough, he was arrested for attempting to shoplift.

Mom and I went to visit Jerry behind bars. The jail was dark and dank, smelling like mouldy socks mixed with urine. I saw him behind the bars, and felt my stomach wrench. He looked so pathetic now; not such a cool hardcore biker dude after all. Mom promised him she would get him out of that hellhole in no time, gave him a kiss through the bars, and we headed back out into the sunshine and fresh air.

I never saw Jerry again. Sheila later told me that he was killed on his Harley Davidson. I imagine most of Mom's friends killed themselves one way or another long before their time was truly up.

Chapter 11

All play and not much work

Mom did various jobs to make ends meet. In Massachusetts she worked at a large industrial factory as a manual labourer, then as an Avon representative, and later was a bar maid in the evenings where she quite often took us to work with her. She wore her white Go-Go boots, a short white mini skirt and backcombed her dark shoulder length hair into a beehive. Her eyes were heavily made up with black eye liner and mascara, and her lips were pale.

While Mom served drinks behind the bar, Sheila and I liked to hang out and play pool. Sometimes when it was busy we asked the patrons if they would give us a quarter — promising we would sing and dance for them. We dropped the quarter into the Jukebox, hit the button for 'All Shook Up' and ran to the stage for our performance. We shook our legs singing along and were met with rapturous cheer at the end of the song. Many nights were spent like this instead of being in bed. It was all part of a normal day, or more accurately night, and life for us.

When Mom wasn't working, which was more often than not, she was partying. Once during a night of heavy drinking, she and her friends thought it would be funny to get me drunk. I was getting lots of positive attention, so I continued to swig a bottle of whiskey to entertain them. The last thing I remember was lying on my back on my bed choking on my own vomit and being too drunk to coordinate my body. My world was swirling around me like water flushing down a toilet bowl. Luckily Sheila had enough sense to roll me over to stop me from choking to death. In the morning, I awoke in a puddle of my own cold stinking vomit.

A few nights later and I was showing off amongst Mom's friends while she slept on the couch. I was saying, 'Fucking assholes. You're shit. Fuck you. Bastards!' Imagine my surprise when Mom walked up behind me and hit me very hard on the head with a large metal spoon. In embarrassment, I retreated to Sheila's and my little room. I sat on the bed, placed my elbows on my knees and held my head in my hands, sulking, looking at the floor. It was then that I noticed blood spurting out the top of my head. I screamed and Mom rushed in to find my blood everywhere.

Mom reluctantly took me to a nearby hospital. Whilst lying on the doctor's table, the doctor asked me how I had cut my head, and I wet myself in fear of what may happen if I told the truth. Mom looked at me with a cold hard stare that told me I was dead if I said it. I didn't know what else to say — I wasn't a rehearsed liar, so I told the truth. Mom resorted to her favourite leather belt to beat us. That day she gave me ten lashes for telling the truth, and ten lashes for wetting my pants. My bottom was sore for days.

Mom reserved the belt for special occasions, so it wasn't often used on us, especially not on me. Because I was the baby of the family, I evaded a lot more of Mom's emotional and physical abuse than did Sheila or Tina. What would hurt me most, and Mom knew it, was ignoring me and giving me the cold treatment, which is when she acted as if I didn't exist, not speaking to me or acknowledging my presence. Mom also had a quick temper and we were weary of her backhand that came flying at us out of nowhere -whacking us hard across the face or head. I would and still do, flinch, duck, and cower at the slightest quick moment in my peripheral vision.

One night whilst Mom and her friends partied, a bum fell asleep with a lit cigarette in the corridor outside our door. Nobody noticed that the air was hot, dry and stunk like a barbeque until the lights flickered and went out. Through the crack at the bottom of our front door I could see the fire burning brightly on the other side. We retreated to our windows, realising when we opened them there was no fire escape. As if by an act of God, there just happened to be a fire station two buildings down from us, so the brigade were with us within minutes, evacuating us through the windows of the second story building.

The bum who started the fire turned out to be the brother of one of Mom's friends, who up to this point had never made claim. Unfortunately, the bum didn't make it out alive. His brother did. Mom, my sisters and I, and some strange people were temporarily re-homed in Hotel Tropicana for a couple of nights before we moved to Hotel California, so affectionately named by Mom.

Chapter 12

Hotel California

Hotel California was an old condemned hotel offering exceptional views of parking lots, garbage bins, and dumped furniture. Infested with cockroaches, smelling of urine, and inhabited by the homeless, this was our new place for the next few months.

The first thing I did when we saw our room was head for the kitchen. I tugged with all my weight on the large chrome handle of the 50's style fridge. Inside there was an enormous white cockroach that had obviously never seen daylight staring back at me as equally unimpressed as I was. It had been feeding on a broken egg, the only other occupant inside the fridge. With time I became accustomed to cockroaches. Indeed, I was soon playing with them as most children do a hamster.

Standing in the middle of the room, the first thing I saw was a double window looking down on a few skips behind Sears department store. To the right of the windows was a small kitchen about three by four feet. I was standing in the one room that would serve as dining room, lounge, and bedroom, and there was a small bathroom on the right hand side of the room. The walls were a bile tinted grey from years of soot and cigarette smoke. I could see where old posters and pictures had once hung, their white shadows left behind. This place did have a cool bed that folded up into the wall, which was where Tina, Sheila and I slept or were folded up into when Mom wanted some space. Mom would sleep on a single bed across the room against the wall.

It was whilst living at Hotel California that Tina came home again. I loved when Tina was around. She was always so happy, and because she was older I always saw her as a parental figure and felt much more secure in her presence. She gave me lots of kisses and cuddles, helped me make things to eat, reminded me to shower and change my clothes. She was the only one, too, that would question Mom when she was getting out of control. This was good for Sheila and me, but got Tina into a lot of scrapes. Tina was old enough to question 'why?' and Mom didn't like it. She was also old enough to be a physical match to Mom, and this became a problem in that Mom was running out of options on how to handle her daughter who was quickly becoming a young woman with a mind of her own. Unfortunately as a result, not long after Tina returned, Mom kicked Tina out and sent her away.

Sitting in the front seat of Mom's car, we drove over a fly-over in Santa Rosa. Mom pointed to a place below where there were a load of sleeping bags and cardboard boxes on the ground and said, 'That's where Tina lives now.' I swallowed hard and wondered why Mom had sent her away to such a horrible place. I loved my sister and didn't understand why Mom was so mean to her. I didn't reply; I was hoping my silence would have the same sobering effect on her as hers had on me.

After Tina was gone, Mom continued to party day and night. Sometimes she even got Sheila and me involved. One night they put my kitten into a brown paper bag, blew in lungs full of marijuana smoke, and spun the poor kitten around finally letting it go on the floor. I felt deeply pained as I watched the kitten zigzag across the floor desperately trying to get away, but Mom and her friends were in fits of laughter. Next my sister and I played cards with them and if we lost we had to do something one of them suggested. I lost twice. The first time I had to put a large pan over my head, take a metal serving spoon, go up and down the corridor outside our room banging the pot loudly saying, 'Pussy for sale!… Pussy for sale!' I thought it was funny and was getting lots of attention, so I continued to bang and advertise that my pussy was for sale. The more they laughed, the more I banged and advertised.

The second time I lost I had to put my head in the toilet bowl whilst Mom flushed it. Even though they were still laughing, I didn't find it fun anymore and didn't want to play after that.

Whilst living in Hotel California, Sheila and I got up, dressed and went to school and back each day. That Halloween the school held a massive party in the auditorium and all students were invited but had to dress in costume to attend. Sheila and I really wanted to go, but Mom had no money to spare from her drinking allowance so we improvised. I took a tea towel and put it over my head and said to Sheila that I was Little Red Riding Hood, and Sheila took one of Mom's bandannas, wrapped it around her head and said she was a Hell's Angel motorcyclist.

It was early evening and we were on our own when we showed up in our makeshift costumes. It was the only party either of us had been to, so when we walked into the auditorium I was taken aback by the decorations that hung from ceiling to floor. I stood on my own relishing all the sparkly magic and charm. The hall was packed with shrills of laughter as hoards of young children enjoyed themselves. They felt no fear, no insecurities. The happiness around me not only hurt, but also frightened me. Happiness like this was something I didn't understand. Watching the genuine display of trust and willingness to engage, I was painfully aware for the first time in my life how dirty and utterly alone I felt. I believed I didn't belong.

When we weren't at school, Sheila and I liked to look through the local mall's waste bins salvaging broken lamps and other expensive artefacts. We also regularly raided the local Goodwill boxes where other people deposited goods they no longer wanted. Once we pulled open the door of a Goodwill box and slid through the small opening at the top. We were frantically going through what we could find, fighting over whom got what when a passer by stopped and knocked on the outside, 'Anybody in there?'

'No,' we both replied at the same time and sat quietly thinking that playing dead would make the passer by move on. They didn't, which as it happened was a good thing. Helped out by a very nice looking middle-aged man, we were quizzed as to why we were in there in the first place. Sheila said we had dropped a toy inside by mistake and we were looking for it. Giving us food tokens from his pocket, he warned us not to do it again and sent us on our way.

One day before Mom had sent Tina away again, I went out on my own to the local Wal-Mart store with an empty handbag draped over my shoulder. I walked systematically up and down the isles filling the bag with things like socks, underwear, shampoo, toothpaste, hairbrushes and clips. With the bag completely stuffed full, I headed for the door. On the way out, I saw a tin of band-aids and grabbed that too, but because the bag was already full, I just held it in my hands and exited.

As I headed back to Hotel California, two members of staff from the store ran after and stopped me. They wanted to see what was in my bag but I wouldn't let them. Instead I ran all the way back to Mom. The staff members followed and spoke with Mom explaining that I had been shoplifting. Mom agreed to let them take me back to the store for interrogation. She didn't come with me — Tina did. Once the staff heard why I had stolen all the goods, that we had nothing at home, they gave me a warning, an affectionate look, a pat on the back, and told me to go home. In retrospect, if the same thing were to happen today the authorities would be called in to find out why we had nothing at home.

In front of Hotel California there was a second hand shop that my sisters and I would regularly browse, eyes wide-open and mouths drooling. It's amazing how one person's junk is another person's treasure. On my own one day I found a cute bright red vinyl coin purse that cost 10 cents. I didn't have 10 cents, so I stole it. Back at home I showed Sheila and she said, 'You stole that!'

'No, I didn't!' I protested, 'I searched the gutters and found 10 cents.'

'No you didn't 'cause I already looked and there wasn't any money there!'

Chapter 13

I love you too Mommy

Mom allowed Tina to come home again after we moved to a new place behind a seedy bar. It looked like the Bates Motel from the movie Psycho with the exception that attached to one end was a chicken shed. That was my sisters' and my room. At night we bedded on the shelves using anything we could find to keep warm and Mom put a padlock on the door so that nobody could get in, and more importantly nobody could get out.

One stormy evening, Mom had forgotten to lock us in, and the door was slamming open and shut from the force of the wind. Rain gusted through the door and leaked through the ceiling onto my sleeping bag. Lightening illuminated the shed and thunder rumbled the shelf I was lying on. Frightened, wet and cold, I went outside and into Mom's room next door, which was more like a shack, with a kitchenette, a closet with no door, a room with a shower and sink, and a floor – which is more than our shed had. She was asleep in her single bed and I didn't dare wake Mom so I huddled myself in the chair at her feet. I was freezing but felt safe near her so remained there in a ball as if a cat curled in on itself trying to keep warm.

Mom woke in the night and found me asleep in the chair. Instead of being cuddled and reassured, Mom heavily scolded and took me hastily back to the chicken shed. This time the lock was not forgotten. I climbed into Tina's sleeping bag and snuggled her for reassurance and a source of warmth.

The following morning we couldn't get out to use the loo because Mom was still asleep. I could see the weather had changed by the sun beaming through the cracks in the ceiling and wooden slatted door. Peering through a gap, I looked out at the gravel parking lot in front. Patrons and residents parked their rusty Ford pick up trucks and Pintos, and judging from how full the lot was, it was around 11:00 am. That's when the bar started to fill up each day.

When Mom finally opened our door there was no warm breakfast waiting for us; she had no food to feed us. We stayed outside in the lot to play and stayed well clear of Mom. Sometimes we went on adventures in search of food – like the time we found a field of corn. We peeled back the husks and sank our teeth into the raw cobs filling our bellies so quickly we made ourselves sick.

It was at this place that Sheila and I started a game called the Peacock Race, which was basically tag but we had to act like peacocks doing it. The idea was in memory of the house in the Redwoods Mom had promised us; it was there we had seen peacocks for the first time. We looked more like chickens with our heads cut off as we flapped our wings (elbows), bent our legs into a squatting position and frantically chased one another around the parked cars.

Full of excitement, we bound into Mom's room to tell her about our new game. She was watching a soap opera and wanted us to 'get lost.' We didn't. Instead, we sat at her feet giggling and whispering to each other. Without warning, Mom jumped up, grabbed me by the waist, carried me outside under her arm to the industrial size garbage bin, opened the heavy metal lid, put me in and shut the lid again. She then went for Sheila who thought it was a marvellous game, running away from her in fits of giggles. Mom caught and scooped Sheila up too, placing her inside the bin with me, and closing the lid once again. Willing to take any form of attention we could get, we shared in Mom's laughter as once again Sheila and I were looking at each other inside a garbage bin.

My sisters and I had many unconventional ways of entertaining ourselves, ranging from playing at the local car junkyard, to scouting out old warehouses and buildings, ripping out colourful wires from their electrical boxes and making bracelets and rings by twisting them together. On one of our daily adventures we found a dead roof rat, which was about the size of a small cat, took it home and played with it for hours. We put it in a shoebox, used a tea towel to cover it like a blanket, and spoke to it like a baby. This is what happened when we didn't have toys to play with – we improvised.

The only toy we did have was a Grover puppet. Grover was our favourite Sesame Street character, so when we found the puppet at a second hand shop, we didn't mind that his red bulbous nose was half missing, or that his blue fur was dirty and matted. Poor abandoned Grover needed love, and we were just the girls to give it to him. First we sympathetically repaired his nose by stuffing it with pink toilet paper. Then we spent hours and hours talking to him, and him talking to us. Sheila was always the puppeteer bringing him to life by mimicking one of our favourite sketches, 'A Waiter's Memory':

'Yes Sir! Grover at your service, Sir! You is my only pleasure, Sir!' said Grover while I snuggled into Sheila's side and giggled.

'Sir! I am a trained professional. I do not need to write things down. Instead I use my waiter's memory.'

I adlibbed what the diner said next and asked, 'Well yeah, but I ordered a cheeseburger with French fries and a pickle. Isn't that a lot to remember?'

'Ha!' said Grover. 'Observe, Sir – a trick of the trade. I remember things with a little poem. Listen: *Round and tasty on a bun – pickles, French fries, yum yum yum.'*

'How are you going to remember it's for me?' I asked giggling in anticipation of his answer.

'Ummm, OK: *In a hurry to be fed, beady eyes and big blue head. HA HA!'*

Sheila and I loved that bit. Every time Grover said it we laughed like it was the first time we had heard it. Good ol' Grover was so much fun and he only cost us a quarter.

It was whilst living at the Bates Motel that Mom woke me in the night. She kissed me, told me she loved me and said goodbye. I looked at her through sleepy eyes and said, 'I love you too Mommy,' and fell back to sleep thinking nothing more of it. In the morning, she was nowhere to be found but had left a note with a telephone number of an ex-boyfriend for us to ring. Tina was once again living in another group home, so it was Sheila who sacrificed her cherished last dime to use the pay phone outside the local seedy boozer. I don't recall the conversation; I just know that within 45 minutes a Social Service Worker had shown up at our door.

When she explained to us that she had to take us away to somewhere safe, trying to escape from the pending doom, we ran outside and into the bar. It was early in the day, again around

11:00 am, and the bar was already heaving with local drunks whom we knew quite well. We ran and hid under their legs, hoping the Social Worker would give up and leave us alone.

With the help of some of the patrons we were dragged out of the bar kicking and screaming and taken to Mom's room. The Social Worker, Suzanne, desperately tried to talk sense to us and explain why we couldn't possibly stay there on our own, but Sheila shouted with all the fight she could muster, 'There's a roof over our heads; I can make corn bread to eat. We're fine! Leave us alone. I can look after Lora – always have…'

Chapter 14

Dependent unit

Despite our reasonable protests and obvious ability to look after ourselves, we were re-homed. Social Services weren't really sure what to do with us at this point; didn't know if Mom would show up again and want custody, or if we were disturbed due to our circumstances. As a result, we were placed in the Dependant Unit (DU) on the outskirts of Santa Rosa in the countryside. The building consisted of two large halls on either side of a central building; one for the boys, one for the girls and a central meeting ground in the middle. There were about 60 of us in total, 30 in each block. We each had our own room with a single bed and cupboard for our belongings, and shared a large communal toilet block with showers. The DU catered for ages ranging from infant to eighteen, but when I was there the ages ranged from five to sixteen. It was actually the nicest place I had ever stayed over night. It was certainly very different from the cockroach infested Hotel California, or the smelly chicken shed we had just been sleeping in.

When Sheila and I arrived, Tina was already there having failed at her previous group home. Tina tucked me under her wing, protected me from some of the older girls, and continued to care for me as a mother would her daughter. It would be the last time for many years that us three girls were together again.

I learned many things during my stay at the DU. First I learned to volunteer to tidy up the clothes cupboard. This ensured I got the clothes I wanted to wear by hiding them whilst I tidied. My favourite outfit was a pair of red bell-bottom cords and a white long sleeve button up shirt. Both were a little big, but I liked the swishing sound the cords made when I walked, and the shirt went well with the cords. Not only that, but they looked like what Tina wore and I liked that.

Although there were several other children I could have played with at the DU, I always preferred the attention of the staff because it was one of the first times in my life I was receiving positive attention from which I could grow and learn. One staff member, Marty, a man in his late 20's with thick black shoulder length hair and a full beard, took me for evening walks. We would talk about nothing in particular, just things. On the way back to the centre, he would challenge me to a race, promising me if I won I could have custard from the kitchen. Each evening he would let me almost win, and then overtake me at the last second. He still let me have custard, though.

Another staff member, Laura, let me help cook simple treats like chocolate chip cookies. In fact, it was because of her encouraging my interests in food that I developed a real flair for cooking and baking that would remain with me until the present day. It was a way of controlling and mastering something that previously I had no influence over.

On other occasions, a group of children and I were taken in a large van to the ocean, a forty-five minute drive away. On the way we would sing *99 Bottles of Beer on the Wall* and *American Pie* by Don McLean. They brought us to a place Mom used to take my sisters and me called Goat Rock, where we made sand candles, hunted for crabs and starfish and ate our sandy sandwiches. Visiting places that meant something to Mom made me feel like the umbilical cord that had connected her to me was still pumping life between us. As I stood in the cold wind looking out at the large rock island with goats on top, I pictured Mom beside me, sharing my love and pain the way only she could.

Back at the DU in the central building, there was a communal area with couches, beanbags, and chairs for the children to sit and watch TV. The staff's office had large windows facing inwards over the communal area so they could keep watch. In another part of the central block, there was a large pool table and dartboard, and just off the central building was the kitchen/dining area that looked like a school's canteen. There was also a separate fully equipped baby unit off the central building that wasn't being used where I was allowed to play on my own. There was always plenty to do and plenty of people to do it with, so while I waited for Mom to make her reappearance as she always did, I quite enjoyed my time at the Dependent Unit.

Each day, a bus clearly marked with the Sonoma County Social Services logo dropped off and picked me up at a local school. As a result, I made no friends because the logo clearly made me different. At recess and lunch break, I would wander to the end of the playground, sit on the ground leaning against one of the many tall pine trees and watch the other children playing. In class I was quiet but like a sponge I absorbed as much knowledge as I could, learning as quickly as they could teach me. I was the only student who knew the correct meaning and difference between the words 'two, to, and too' and could recognise which one to spell when the teacher said the word in a sentence. Since I was only seven, I felt very proud of myself for this.

There was a teenage boy in the DU who said he might want to be my boyfriend, but it was a toss up between me and another girl. We both had to kiss him and whoever kissed the best would get to be his. I met him around the back of the centre. He was leaning very coolly with his weight pressed against one foot propped up on the wall behind him. I nervously walked up, giggled and fidgeted my fingers. He gave me permission to stand before him. I took my place, sucked in a deep breath, closed my eyes, puckered my lips, leaned in and gave him a peck on the mouth – then turned and quickly ran away. The other girl kissed him using her tongue, so she became his girlfriend. I had stood no chance, but no great love lost. I still thought a guy was only good to party with or be abandoned by.

Not only did I learn that you should kiss boys using your tongue, I also proved myself to be a hot little pool-player. The staff held a pool competition between a load of teenage guys and me — the only girl. I got to the semi-finals without much effort and earned myself a respectable reputation amongst the guys. Following the pool tournament, they tucked me under their wings and let me hang out with them. On hot summer days the guys and I hiked into the hilly ridges behind us and hunted for rattlesnakes. When we found one, they used sticks in the shape of a 'Y' to pin the snake's head down while another used his switchblade to cut off the snake's rattler. They gave me one and explained that like the rings on a tree, you can tell how old a rattlesnake is by counting the number of segments or 'rings' it has in its rattler. Mine was eight. Looking back it seems so cruel and dangerous, but at the time it was exhilarating.

When it wasn't rattlesnake hunting, it was catching Blue Belly lizards at an abandoned barn in a field close by. We had to be fast and couldn't grab them by their tail because the lizards detached them to get away. I quickly learned it was best to only catch the little ones – the big ones bite hard! After our fill of lizard hunting, we tried to throw stones up and over the electrical wires outside the DU centre. I never did quite make it, despite the boys' attempts to show me how easy it was.

'You see,' they explained, 'It's easy. Up and over,' as they threw stone after stone over the wire. Not being able to do this was always a real disappointment for me – I was usually so good at keeping up with the guys.

Whilst I forged relationships with others, Tina and Sheila had a break from the role of parenting me, able to be young girls with no responsibilities while somebody else made sure my needs were being met. It was one of the first times where we all felt comfortable enough to stop clinging to each other and start thinking on our own, being our own individual – not part of a unit. All that said, we still had regular meetings in the evening where we would come together in Tina's room, sit on her bed and talk about our day. If I had any problems with any of the other children, I would tell my sisters, confident that by morning the issues would be resolved.

While the staff continued to evaluate our situation wondering what to do with us next, Mom showed up. At this point, some months down the line, I was a ward of the court and we were only allowed to have closely monitored visits with Mom in a small room with only one way in and out. Mom visited us a couple of times, and each visit ended with me hanging onto her leg sobbing and begging her to take me home. I couldn't understand why we couldn't go with her. Yes, she had left us – as she had done many times before – but she was back now; she should be taking us with her when she left.

When it was visiting day again, I couldn't wait to see Mom. In my mind I had been rehearsing for days all the things I wanted to tell her. I had been a good girl and earned points that I was able to buy things with from a shop. One of the things I bought, which I couldn't wait to give her, was a poster of a white horse on a bright pink background. I imagined how pleased she would be because she liked horses.

After waiting anxiously all day, eventually evening came, and I slowly accepted she wasn't coming. I didn't want to play pool or watch TV. I didn't want to eat. My sixth sense knew that she was never coming back. Consumed with sorrow, I walked around with a void in my gut not wishing to laugh or cry — not wishing to be alive at all. Feeling lost and numb, I went to bed early placing the poster carefully under my mattress. In the morning I realised I had wet the bed and it had destroyed the poster below.

I cut the imaginary umbilical cord between Mom and me and started telling people that she was dead – that was why she wasn't there for me. I later learned from Mom that according to her version of the story, she had lost permanent custody and couldn't bear facing us again. I don't think it works quite like that. I believe, in fact, they give the mother many opportunities to redeem herself. She never even tried. She took the easy route out.

The next morning at school, standing in the back row of chorus with my classmates singing, 'She sails away, on a happy summer's day, on the back of a crocodile,' I suddenly felt violently ill. I raised my hand but couldn't get the words out that I was feeling unwell before I had been sick everywhere. Taken back to the Dependent Unit, I remained in bed for a week. Apparently they could find nothing wrong with me.

Chapter 15

A mere parcel

For the next couple of years I surfed the social service system in Sonoma County. For a couple of months they tried keeping Sheila and me together, but in the end when we were placed with a family that decided Sheila was a bad influence over me, we were separated.

On a hot summer's day, standing on the pavement of a street lined with trees, everything in me ached as I watched my sister, my best friend, slowly driven away from me. For the first time in my life I experienced a deadening of my soul. The very last thing that meant something to me was being taken away. Feelings were no use to me anymore – I didn't need them. All I could feel now was a ruthless anger pumping blood through me. I tightened my lips as once again I was being treated as if I were a mere parcel with no say over my destination.

Sitting on the back seat of the car, Sheila turned and pressed the palm of her hand on the window. One of a few true moments of my ability to fight was upon me. In this brief instant, I retreated and built a huge brick wall around my heart. I was not a victim. I was safely inside – a sea of emotion frozen in stone. Nobody could get to me in here. I would never be the same person again.

I was used to Tina not being there, but Sheila had been my constant companion and suddenly without that security, I felt vulnerable and alone like a misplaced piece of puzzle. I was always tired and ill; my tummy cramped and I couldn't concentrate on the simplest of things because I was too busy in my head thinking about what had happened.

The couple that took me into their home wanted to make me something I wasn't. First the lady of the house permed my straight blond hair and made it curly like a poodle's coat. Then she replaced all my comfortable 'Tom Boy' clothes with expensive itchy dresses. I was constantly reminded of my manners, how to sit, speak, and eat. I felt on edge, like I was acting out a role in somebody else's play and didn't want to forget my lines. I was still myself on the inside, though. I was always constant and true to myself even when others tried to deceive. I was not easily misled and confused. I knew my own mind and they were not allowed in. They could not poison me with their toxic garbage. I was better than that.

Outside they had a mermaid water feature with large lily pads. Deep in imagination, I waded in, took the lily pads and laid them at the mermaid's feet. I then went and found a snail and placed it on the lily pads. I truly did not realise this would bring them harm, but when the lady of the house saw what I had done she became irate, ranting that the lily pads were from some exotic place in the world and irreplaceable. Within a week, I was back at the DU: this parcel once again returned to sender.

Chapter 16

The Grists

Not long after I was returned to the DU, they shipped me off to a new place with The Grists, Lucille and Roland, an elderly couple whose daughter had grown and moved out years before.

The Grists were in their mid sixties and strict Seventh Day Adventists. This meant I was only allowed to watch television if it was the news, and Saturdays — following church service — were spent resting all day on my bed, which is really difficult when you are 8. They were kind people, but old, so they found my energy challenging. I felt like Dennis the Menace who continually and accidentally wound up the elderly next-door neighbour. My curiosity and lack of experience got me into constant trouble, like the time I picked buckets full of plums from the orchard behind their house. Seeing how happy Mrs Grist was, and wanting to please her even more, I took it one step further and washed them in her large laundry sink with very hot soap and water. When all the plums went off in the heat, I asked Mrs Grist what was wrong with them, and she nearly pulled her white hair out in frustration. I had ruined all the jars of jam that she would have sold to a local shop as she did each year.

Mr Grist read the bible in his living room wingback chair almost all day every day, while Mrs Grist practised next week's church hymns on her organ. I would sit next to her and sing, 'Give me oil in my lamp, keeping me burning. Give me oil in my lamp, I pray...' in the most operatic voice I could, and Mrs Grist would say to her husband who sat quietly reading in the corner, 'Isn't her singing lovely, dear?'

The Grists had lived in the same house on the same street all of their married lives. They had raised their only daughter there, now in her early thirties, and planted the small orchard behind their house. The home was so well established and secure that every piece of furniture and artwork looked like it existed just to fill that spot in their home. The only thing that seemed out of place was me.

When I first moved in with the Grists there were two other foster children: Jill, age 17, and Becky, 18. I don't know what circumstances led them to living with the Grists, but I could tell from our first meeting that neither of them was all there upstairs. Jill was tall, bone thin, nervous, had shoulder length greasy brown hair, and was covered in spots. Becky was a lesbian and soon after I arrived left the Grists to join the army. She had a short back and sides haircut, wore vests to show off her masculine arms and tattoos, and acted like most men I had met except I liked her; she was very nice to me. It didn't matter me what her sexual preference was, but it definitely bothered the Grists who continually reminded Becky that she was going to hell.

There was such an age difference between me and the other foster children I didn't quite know what to do with myself. If I wasn't outside making mud patties and stepping on their cats' tails for fun, I was spending long hours in my room pretending to be a strict teacher, writing on the chalkboard that hung on the door of my closet. I applied the sample deep red Avon lipstick that Mrs Grist had given me, and held a wooden yardstick that I repeatedly beat the imaginary students with when they got an answer wrong.

One day after I became bored of being the strict teacher, I sat on the end of my bed wondering what to do next. I wasn't accustomed to being alone all the time. On a whim, I decided I wanted to scare Jill. I took her watch from her room and a plastic spider from mine, and strategically placed them just under the edge of her bed so that when she looked and reached for her watch, she would see a spider out of the corner of her eye and think it was real. It worked too; she screamed so loud the windows shook. I didn't tell her I had done it to scare her, and held back an evil grin as she tried to collect herself. I thought how proud Sheila would have been of me, and as my inner smile faded, I asked myself 'now what?'

On other days, I did more fun things like loitering in a funeral home in a room full of resting corpses while Mrs Grist talked to the Funeral Director about which songs to play on the organ during an upcoming ceremony.

The room was hexagonal, and each wall was covered in a deep-blue heavy velour fabric hanging ceiling to floor with an open coffin in front – some occupied, others not. I couldn't work out how to get out of the room, so in my usual style I decided to stand and wait for the situation to sort itself.

Curious what a dead person looks like, I wandered tentatively over to one of the open caskets and looked inside. The beautiful woman lying before me didn't look dead. She looked like she was maybe 50 years old with backcombed black hair. She had bright red lips and an eerie calm expression on her face. Her snow-white skin had finely etched lines making her look fragile and exquisite like a porcelain doll. Her slender hands rested gently folded across her breasts. Her fingernails were a bright scarlet red to match her lips. She looked to me like an older version of Sleeping Beauty. I felt extremely moved and spoke to her in my mind. I asked her if she was OK, was she happy? I told her she was lucky – she didn't have to suffer anymore. I asked her where she was, was it a better place than where she had been in life?

When Mrs Grist finally came to collect me, I felt sad to leave Sleeping Beauty. I said goodbye and wished her well. In retrospect, I understand that the woman in the casket represented Mom. I was saying goodbye to Mom, believing she really was dead.

Later that year, the Grists took me to a large Seventh Day Adventists conference in Salt Lake City, Utah. I was left in a large room with about thirty other children and felt painfully shy. Usually Sheila would have protected and given me more confidence, but now I was exposed and on my own. The adults were asking us difficult questions about characters and incidents from the Bible.

Oh, please don't ask me.... Please don't, my thoughts were interrupted by a question.

'And what do you think he built his house on – sand or stone?' asked an overly perky look-alike mannequin.

Sand sounded good. I like sand. 'Sand' I answered.

Everybody, including the adults, laughed at me and I shrank inwardly thinking how much I hated God if this was what he was all about.

I don't know if it was because the Grists were so religious, but I used to see faceless angels surrounding my bed at night. They never spoke or moved they just bowed their heads over me and wore white robes. Frightened to breathe deeply or move in case they would physically touch me, I would lay motionless until I fell asleep. Once I found the energy around me so overwhelming I decided I couldn't take it anymore. I plucked up enough courage and bounded out of my bed. I ran to Mrs Grist in tears, and she made me a root beer float. As I slurped down the soda and ice cream through a straw, she explained very kindly that I was lucky to have so many angels looking over me. She promised me they would never hurt me. They were there to protect me. After that, I didn't mind them so much.

Not long after and without any warning, the Grists took me out of school one day to go see a doctor. I spoke with the doctor, and then waited while the Grists spoke to him in private for an equal length of time. When they came out of his office, we silently got into their mint green Lincoln Mercury and drove for quite a while. To my horror, I suddenly recognised where we were. I sat stunned and mortified hoping this wasn't what I thought it was. The car was making its way up the long tree lined road that led to the Dependent Unit.

The Grists remained quiet as we pulled up. They unloaded two suitcases of my belongings as I sat and watched silently. They took me inside, and I waited in the same room I used to visit Mom. I was in there on my own for about twenty minutes when a member of staff collected me, brought me to a room, and told me to unpack my things. Nobody ever spoke to me about why I was returned to the DU. The Grists never even said goodbye. I felt completely unloved, misunderstood, and alone in a cruel world. I really didn't and still don't know what I had done to deserve being returned once again.

Apparently now labelled disturbed, I was subsequently placed in a Group home run by an organisation called Children's Garden.

Great, now I had a reputation as being disturbed. I didn't feel disturbed. I felt like I was the only sane person around. I was in one of the organisation's homes for a while where I was being home schooled with the other children, obviously too disturbed to mix with other human beings, when suddenly for some reason I was shipped off to another Group home being run by Bob and Carolyn Boynton.

Chapter 17

The Boyntons

Bob and Carolyn were both twenty-six when I met them. What struck me most was how outgoing and dynamic they were. Bob was attractive in a Luke Skywalker from Star Wars young boy kind of way. He stood 5' 9", had warm brown eyes that twinkled and smiled, light brown hair, and an open kind face. Carolyn was a vivacious take-charge kind of gal. If you wanted something done efficiently, she was your woman. She was short, standing at 5'1", also had warm brown eyes, and her deep, rich brown hair was short and sassy. I could see why many men either appreciated and were drawn to her fiery, outgoing nature – or were completely repelled by her domineering ways and ran a million miles in the opposite direction. She ran a tight ship, making sure every last detail in running the household had been well thought out.

I really liked the home I shared with Bob and Carolyn. I never considered any of my other destinations really a home, but this place definitely was. There were seven children including myself. All around my age, there was Marion (really weird), Abe (a black boy who had been locked in a cupboard most of his childhood), David L. (just completely out there), Robbie (eventually medically diagnosed as being psychotic), Ahimsa (a genuinely very nice but slightly disturbed boy), and David C. (who I got on best with).

My fondest memory in this home is of the trips David C. and I made to the top of the hills behind our house. We would set out first thing on numerous summer mornings to hike the steep golden hills that were dotted with grand oak trees, craggy rocks and the odd meandering stream.

It took us the better part of a day to reach the summit where we sat silently throwing pebbles down, appreciating the fantastic views of the green valley full of homes below. We shared the scene with blue skies, wild deer, and circling eagles before devouring the lunch Carolyn had packed for us. The air was hot, smelling like baking dusty earth, but the thin breeze cooled our sweaty skin. We were experiencing internal peace in all its quiet glory.

Full of food and life, we'd had our fill and slowly made our way back down the hill stopping only briefly from time to time to take in shade from an oak, or to search for obsidian carved Indian Head arrows. When we arrived at the bottom of the hill, the day was already drawing in on itself. We ate dinner with Bob, Carolyn, and the other children, feeling a great sense of accomplishment and an unspoken bond between us.

Built on a slope, most of the useable space in our house was upstairs with only one bedroom downstairs. That was my bedroom. It was immediately opposite the front entrance to the house. I never told Bob and Carolyn this, but I was petrified to be on my own so far separated from everybody else. I was terrified that somebody would come through the front door and kidnap me, so night after night I crawled into my closet, sleeping there until morning so that when 'he' did come to get me, 'he' wouldn't be able to find me.

All the children in the Group home had a portrait taken with Bob and Carolyn, and one day I found Bob laying on the floor in the lounge staring at the portrait in deep thought. I lay down next to him, digging my elbows into the shabby mustard coloured carpet, propping my head up on my hands. 'Whatcha thinking about Bob?' I asked.

He breathed in deeply through his nose and said, 'Oh, I'm just looking at all your beautiful faces.'

I liked Bob. He was the first man in my life I trusted. Bob once told me that he knew a week after I arrived in their home I was definitely not disturbed. To him I was just a kid who had a bad break in life and deserved something good to come along.

I liked Carolyn too; she was pretty, funny and her personality glowed. However, she was totally opposite to Mom and this took some getting accustomed to. She was quite outspoken and loud, always busying herself with some chore or another, never slowing down even for an instant. Although she wasn't very affectionate towards me, she made up for it in other ways. When she took me shopping, I was allowed to pick out new clothes for the first time in my life. She even let me pick out a teddy; I chose a fluffy brown monkey with an enormous smile on his face and Velcro on its hands that stuck to his feet. I called him Tickle Toes. For several years he went everywhere with me.

Carolyn also took us to the library a lot, which I adored. I never knew books could be so fascinating. I wasn't so much interested in typical children's books as I was in checking out book after book on Elvis Presley. I would sit outside the library beside a beautiful lake studying all of the photographs of Elvis. When I had my fill of staring at him, I would find peace in sitting quietly watching reflections on the rippled water. I knew I was safe and happy; I appreciated the moments I could slow down, reflect, and be grateful for the place I was at.

After living with them for a year or so, Bob and Carolyn took me to a local park one day, just us, which alerted me straight away that something was underfoot. As I sat on a bench, Bob got down on one knee in an act of proposal and asked me what I would like most from a family. I thought about it for a good few seconds and said, 'A horse.'

Bob chuckled and said, 'Well, we can't say you'll have a horse, but how would you feel about becoming our daughter?'

It was the summer of 1979 when I accepted Bob and Carolyn's proposal. It was and would remain one of the most important days in my life, one I would never forget and for which I am eternally grateful.

Chapter 18

My new family

The home we lived in with the other children belonged to the organisation Children's Garden, so part of moving on and becoming a family meant leaving behind the house and other children I had grown close to. The first thing we did together as a new family, even before moving into our new house, was take a trip to Yosemite National Park. It was winter and I had a debilitating cold. I couldn't breathe through my nose, my head ached, my eyes were watering, and my body felt like one throbbing ache.

We arrived in the evening, and following dinner in a local restaurant, we walked around taking in the starry night. There was a lit outdoor ice-skating rink with children and adults bundled in mittens, scarves, and hats skating round with rosy cheeks and runny noses. Carolyn asked me if I would like to have a go, and normally I would have jumped at the chance, but because I felt so rotten I declined.

Later that evening back at our cabin, I lay in the dark in a single bed across the room from Bob and Carolyn trying to sleep, but I couldn't because I could barely breathe. I kept coughing, snuffling, and moaning when Carolyn finally snapped at me impatiently, insisting I be quiet. I thought, *this isn't what I had in mind for a mother*. I knew that Mom had never been much better, but I thought because I had chosen Carolyn to fill the mother's role, she would embrace it full heartedly and know exactly what to do. I didn't understand that she had never done the job before, and what's more, I always had an unwarranted feeling it was Bob who wanted to adopt me – not her.

Following our trip to Yosemite, and before moving into our new home, Bob took me to his mother's house for a night in San Francisco. It was a lovely comfortable home and Bob enjoyed telling me all about his childhood spent there. His family home, originally built on Treasure Island in the middle of San Francisco Bay as the 'House of the Future,' was rebuilt on the mainland, and looked very different from the other Victorian properties around. For a start, there were two front entrances, and it was only single-story. That night I learned his father had died when he was only seventeen, that his grandfather, Albert E. Boynton, had been the State Senator of California twice, and that he had one older sister, Mimi.

Aunt Mimi recently wrote me an email about their mom and dad:

> *My mother was a saint, but my father was an old drunken tyrant who had me in tears 5 nights out of 7 at the dinner table. Bob disappeared from the fray and dinked around in his room, the invisible child who grew up without a dad, as a momma's boy who cooked. Could be worse. Nobody grows up unscathed, and maybe we shouldn't grow up in a perfect world. Adversity grows character. But it shouldn't be such a heavy burden to crush us.*

His mother and stepfather weren't home during our visit, so it was the first time Bob, Carolyn and I were alone in a house as a family. With all the attention and fuss aimed at me, I felt special and powerful; I thought this is how it would be, that everything would revolve around making me happy. To my disappointment, after moving into our new home 20 minutes south of San Francisco, it wasn't long before day-to-day life started resembling a more balanced pecking order.

I don't think any one of us knew what to expect once we became a family, but I suspect the reality of it was much different than any of us had imagined. Bob and Carolyn wanted to talk about my feelings a lot, as if this was something that should come naturally, but I had a problem with communicating my feelings or needs. Everything was still comfortably numb inside. I had hidden my feelings for so long, I didn't know what or how I should feel.

When I was sitting with Bob on the floor by a furnace outside their bedroom one evening, Bob grabbed me by the shoulders and gently shook me – pleading with me to show some emotion, just say how I was feeling. He was begging me to let the walls down and allow them in. I simply couldn't. Even if I had wanted to, I didn't know how. I feared hurting too much from reconnecting with the pain, or even worse, being abandoned again.

It was enough for me, age nine, finally for the first time in my life to have the stability of a good home with two parents who loved me and who I loved too. Who needed to bring up old feelings anyway? What good could possibly come of it? Although I reasoned myself out of connecting with my emotions, I felt guilty and bad inside that I wasn't the daughter they seemed to want. One day I wrote on my chalkboard, 'I hate myself. I hate myself. I hate myself.' Carolyn came into my room that night as I pretended to sleep and read what I had written. She angrily erased it, mumbling her distaste under her breath. I thought to myself, *now I've done something else to make her hate me.*

Our new home was small, originally a one bedroom house, with a built on room added at the back behind the kitchen; that was my room. Carolyn turned the house into a lovely comfortable home. I had everything a girl could ask for including Barbie dolls, a hamster and a kitten. I enjoyed contributing to the household by vacuuming daily, setting and clearing the table, and doing the dishes. With my weekly allowance, I bought my own cookbooks and tried new recipes by cooking dinner for all of us.

Before becoming a group home parent, Bob put his college degree in music to use by being a band teacher for a high school. Unfortunately, it wasn't long before he realised he hated teaching, especially to doe-eyed adoring teenage girls who only enrolled in band to flirt with him. Being the modest man he is, this kind of behaviour and attention was something he was intensely uncomfortable with. Therefore, Bob had a dilemma when we moved out of the group home: did he go back into teaching, or did he find a new profession? Being an intelligent man, he went to the library and borrowed a few books, studied them and applied for several jobs in computing. One of the first computer companies in the Bay Area hired him and paid a decent salary in return.

I know Carolyn went to college, that's where she met Bob, but I don't know what she studied or what her special interests were. All I know is that there wasn't much she couldn't do when she put her mind to it; therefore, it wasn't difficult for her to find another job working as an assistant at a school that cared for severely disabled children. Like Bob, she borrowed a book and before long, she and I learned sign language. I can still sign the alphabet and ask simple questions like, 'Can you play today?'

It was through frequently visiting Carolyn's work that I learned a great deal of humanity. I will never forget how humbled I was by the severity of some of the children's physical disabilities. There was a black boy around ten years old whose skin hadn't grown since the age of two. The skin on his face was so taut that he couldn't close his eyes, while the skin under them pulled down to his cheekbones, leaving his lower inner bloodied eyelid exposed. One couldn't touch him without breaking his paper-thin skin and causing him to bleed. There were also two brothers, around eight, who had been playing with matches and petrol in their parent's garage when they both caught fire and suffered third degree burns over 90% of their bodies. Their ability to accept their circumstances and still joke and laugh with the staff and me was profoundly moving. They didn't sit questioning, 'Why me?' but rather embraced and found beauty in their world just the way it was. Sometimes even now when I am feeling sorry for myself, I think of those children and find inspiration in their strengths.

It wasn't by mistake that Carolyn gravitated toward care giving roles. She was the eldest child of five and grew up taking on a parental role with her siblings because her mother was a severe alcoholic who also suffered from acute back troubles. This meant Carolyn was in charge of her younger adopted twin brother and sister quite often when her mother was too drunk, hung-over, or in pain to get out of bed.

Carolyn's father was a dentist and was always helping those who had less than they did; he could always be found where he was most needed. The combination of her mother making it necessary and her father who bred it into her as something to be proud of, Carolyn learned to be a caregiver at a very young age; it was a role she was comfortable with and something she knew well. Perhaps this is one of the reasons I struggled to understand why it was so difficult for her in the beginning of our relationship to embrace me as her daughter.

Not long after we moved to San Bruno, I had a nightmare that 'he' was coming to get me. Having awoken in a sweat and floods of tears, I went and knocked on Bob and Carolyn's bedroom door looking for reassurance. Carolyn shouted at me to go back to bed – to stop looking for attention. I was too frightened to go back to my room, so I sat outside their closed door on the floor for about three hours with my arms wrapped around my knees trying to comfort myself. I just wanted her to hug me and say everything would be alright, but instead I felt like I did when I was made to sit on the tyre swing all day in the freezing cold at Uncle Dick's. I could see the warmth emanating from her windows, and wondered why I couldn't be part of the affection and kindness that I knew existed in her.

About six months after we became a family, I tried calling Bob 'Dad' by asking him a question ending it with 'Dad?' He replied, 'Yes DAUGHTER!' in an exaggerated tone. I was so embarrassed at first, but a couple of days later and with a bit of practice, it felt quite natural to call him Dad and Carolyn Mom — and he did, thank God, stop drawing attention to it by saying 'daughter' in return. Within a couple of weeks, I was happily calling my new parents 'Mom and Dad,' and funnily enough, I meant it.

I always believed Mom and Dad's love for me would come naturally. I expected it as most children do from their parents. It never occurred to me that it could be as awkward for them as it was for me. I recently found evidence of this when Mom brought me my old photo albums, scrapbooks, and diaries from that time. In my scrapbook, I found old birthday and Christmas cards from my parents that were signed, *Remember, we 'LOVE' you, Bob 'Dad' and Carolyn 'Mom.'* The words 'LOVE, Dad and Mom' were all in quotes as if they were saying what they felt they should be, but what actually didn't come naturally to them.

I felt closer to Dad because I had never had a father before, or called another man Dad. I trusted him because he was so attentive and sensitive to my needs and he seemed genuinely to like the person I was. I recall looking forward to his bedtime hugs because they were so warm and caring. It was also the time where we would chat about things. Not emotional things, but things like the scientific properties of water and what a strange substance it is, or about God and what we felt Him to be.

On the weekends, Dad would take me on long bicycle rides or to play basketball, but later when I hit puberty and started getting interested in girl things, he found me irritating. It really bothered him that I would run like a girl when we played softball, and he would make fun of the way I spoke mimicking me when I said, 'It's like' and 'totally.' Dad is a perfectionist, so when I started doing things to express my individuality, sometimes questionable things, he couldn't resist the urge to comment in a condescending way, and for a while this drove him and me apart.

Mom and I had a difficult relationship in the beginning. Perhaps it was because I already had a mom once upon a time who I was still hurting over losing, or maybe it was because inevitably I was always comparing. I compared Mom not just against my biological mother but also to the perfect mother I had created in my mind. Quite often she didn't live up to either, and for a long time I couldn't forgive her for that. We seemed to both have our issues and needs, and despite the fact that we desperately wanted to love one another, these needs often created a divide.

Mom couldn't have her own child and so I felt like a constant reminder of that. Ashamedly, I admit I snooped through her journal one day and felt a deep ache behind my ribs as I read, 'Please God, let me have a child of my own. I promise I will even learn to love Lora.' She never knew I read that, and I am sure she will feel terrible when she learns I did, but it is something that happened that made the divide between us even greater for many years.

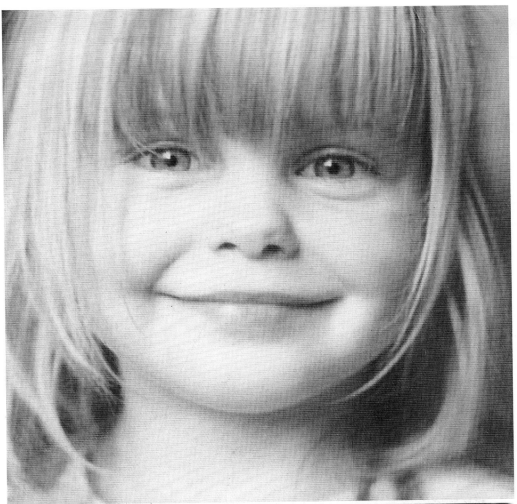

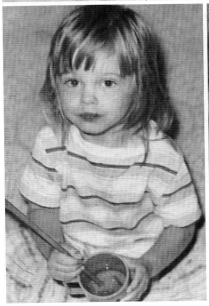

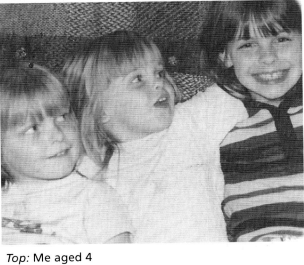

Top: Me aged 4
Left: Me with my favourite cup
Right: Sheila, me and Tina

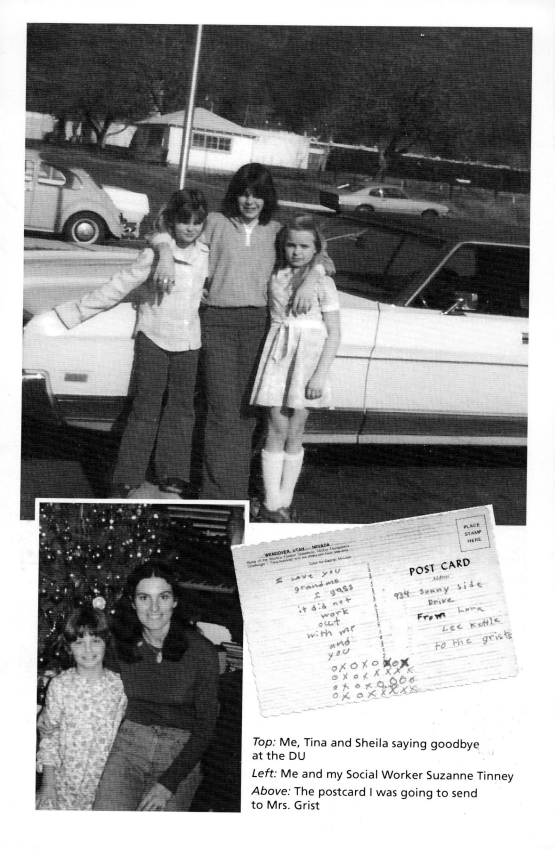

On the postcard:

I love you
grandma
I gass
it did not
work
out
with me
and
you

oxoxo XOX
oxox XXXX
oxoxoooo
oxoxXXXX

POST CARD

Address

934 Sunny side
Drive
From Lora
Lee Kettle
to the grists

Top: Me, Tina and Sheila saying goodbye
at the DU

Left: Me and my Social Worker Suzanne Tinney

Above: The postcard I was going to send
to Mrs. Grist

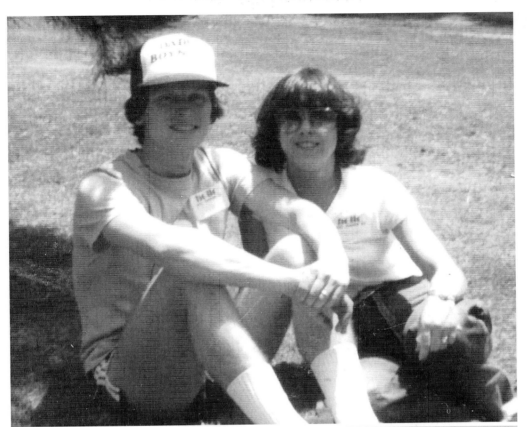

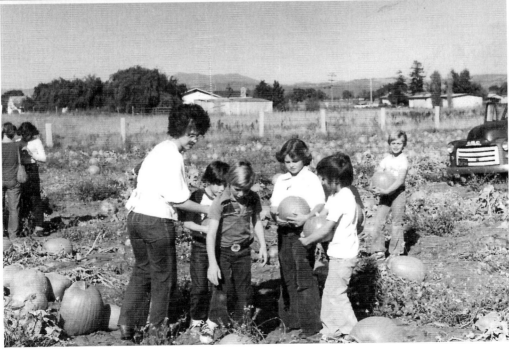

Top: My parents, 1981
Bottom: Searching for the perfect pumpkin—Mom, me and the other group home children

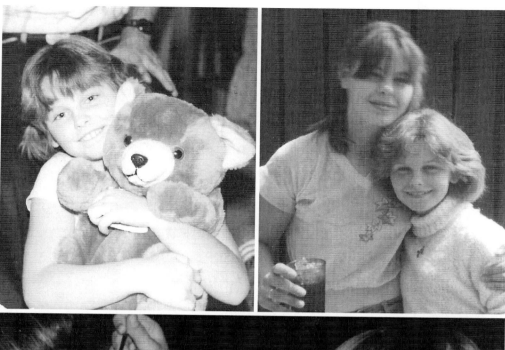

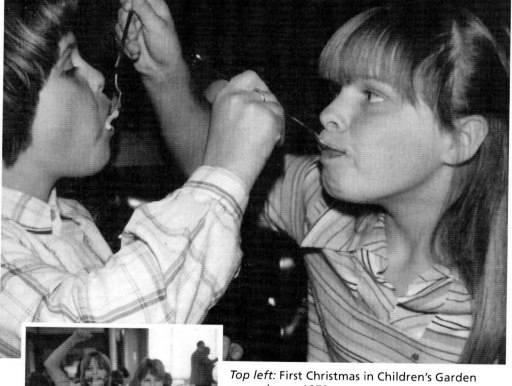

Top left: First Christmas in Children's Garden group home 1979

Top right: Tina and me–First time we had seen each other since the DU

Centre: Me and Sheila–My first birthday with the Boyntons 1980

Left: Sheila and me at a wedding

Whatever our issues were, Carolyn continued to try very hard to care for me like a mother does her child, and it was met with neediness but not necessarily love. I was certainly not all peaches and cream. Sometimes I was mean to her. I resented her trying to control me, as I perceived her efforts of parenting to be. I would often feel glad when she tripped or when she cried. I'm sure she felt the hatred at times, so it's no wonder she found me difficult to love. Overall, I would have too. She never gave up, though, and eventually in our own way we formed a mother-daughter relationship as feeling and complex as you would find in any biologically related mother and daughter. In fact, when I wrote earlier about what Mom is like, I realised for the first time just how much I have turned out so much like her!

Email from Mom

I think about you all the time. Last night Dad & I prayed for you all and talked about the first time we met you. You were eight when we first met you at Children's Garden. We were told to watch for behaviours from you that might appear, like stealing, rebellion, acting out because of the environment you had come from, compounded by abandonment by your mother and separation from your sisters. What we saw was a shy little girl with a beautiful smile who wanted to be accepted. What we remember is a bright girl who wanted to please. You were BY FAR our easiest foster kid. None of the things we were told to watch for happened. You went to school in a regular classroom, we could let you out to play, and you would come back! You were closer to Dad; you never had a father figure before. I remember you enjoyed being a kid, playing, and feeling safe with two parent figures. When we asked you if you wanted us to adopt you, we both remember you replying, 'You are not what I exactly had in mind'. We asked why and you said you always thought your parents would be older and live in the country, more like my parents did. We were 27 years old. Just think 10 years younger than you are now...with no parenting training, criminal really! We muddled through and eventually we became better parents. It was a shock to us at first to be parents at 27 of a 9-year-old girl. I was 30 when you turned 13! But we loved you and were never sad or regretted that we adopted you. I feel God put me on earth to be a Mom to you. I may not have done it well, all the time, but I gave it everything I had. You were my whole life. I never wanted to be anything but a Mom. Really, we all grew up together.

Lora, I love you. I am proud of you. I'm in awe of how well you turned out! You are an amazing woman. Smile sweetie.... Mom

I wasn't the easiest daughter with all my existing problems and issues. What motivated my parents to take on an older child with so many complexities, I will never understand. I can hardly stand when my teenage son acts out, and I have been with him all along his journey. I understand him. My poor parents, at the tender age of 27, took on a thankless mammoth task and got little reward. I started living with them at age 9 and by age 13 I was already pulling away. They didn't get much return on their investment.

Entry from my journal, 5TH August 1983 (13 years old)

Today Mom and I got in a fight – she said I was selfish and a total bitch – she's right though – I feel like I have nobody to talk to anymore. She took my phone away because I was gonna call Shannon and tell her that she couldn't spend the night. I feel so alone in this world. I can't really describe what I'm feeling I'm so frustrated and right now I'm crying. I really love Mom and Dad soooo much – but they don't seem to realize how much I really do love them. I wonder how Mom is feeling right now!! I hope she still loves me. No MATTER what happens, I will ALWAYS LOVE MY MOM and DAD. They just won't love me. Anyway, I just heard my Mom say I'm on restriction. Fuckn' putting me on restriction isn't going to do a fuckn thing except make me mad at them. And to tell you the truth I don't care whether! Or not I'm on restriction doesn't bother me any – so let them think it does – that way there really are not punishing me. Got to go now – Lora.

Chapter 19

Sheila and Tina

Sheila and I were allowed visits over weekends where either I went to stay with her at her foster mom's house two hours away, or she came to stay with us. Waiting for our visits was excruciating. I missed her so much; it meant everything to see her. When my parents started using it as a punishment not to be able to see her if I had been naughty, I felt so angry that other people were giving and taking away things they shouldn't have any power or control over. I felt they shouldn't mess with the relationship shared between sisters, so I retaliated with as much vengeance as I could muster. This usually meant a very bad attitude and tone, or retreating into me altogether and a punishing silent treatment for several days.

When Sheila did visit, she was extremely protective of me so if Mom did or said something to hurt or threaten me, which could be the littlest thing, Sheila would shout at her to leave me alone.

A single woman named Lynn ran Sheila's foster home. I liked Lynn because she did things like take me to Disneyland with my sister and the other five foster children, and always wrote me letters keeping me informed as to what Sheila was up to. What I remember most about Lynn, however, was how obese and lazy she was. She would take us through a Mc Donald's drive through and order us nothing, but get herself four Big Macs. When we got back to her house, she would tell Sheila to come to her room and then demanded Sheila give her a foot massage. Once, we all went on a ten-mile bike ride, and while us children were drenched in sweat trying to get from point A to point B, she rode her moped. Incidentally the moped could barely move under her weight and went slower than we did on our bikes.

I got on well with Sheila's foster brothers and sisters. Like the children from the Group home with Mom and Dad, most of them were disturbed and odd in some way. Like me, Sheila may have been deeply wounded by our past, but was not abnormal or emotionally disturbed. She was, however, aggressive and controlling towards me. Sheila showed her dominance by grabbing my shirt, pulling me towards her then punching me away in the middle of my back as we walked along, or kicking me on my bottom each morning when I lent over to pick up my slippers. Usually I was quite amenable. Up until now, I followed Sheila around like a lost puppy. One day, however, when Sheila tried to treat me badly in front of her foster brothers and sisters, I snapped and fought back.

Sheila's foster siblings gathered around whilst we clawed, punched, bit and pulled each other's hair. Sheila could not afford to lose this fight in front of an audience, and I wasn't backing down, so it took Mom, Dad and Lynn to tear us apart. Once we had calmed down, they wanted to know what had started the fight, but I didn't know how to explain that it was a defining moment, that I was making a statement about my independence and ability to stand up to Sheila, and more importantly, to stand on my own.

On the eighth of July 1983, I found out Sheila was once again living with our biological mother, Terry. Having telephoned her foster home pretending to be a school friend when Lynn answered, Terry asked Sheila if she would like to live with her again in North Carolina. They arranged that Terry would take a Grey Hound bus across the United States and meet her in Rohnert Park. Things didn't go to plan and Sheila was left standing in their designated meeting spot all day before she finally went back to her foster home. It transpired Terry was unable to make their rendezvous because she had been arrested. About a month-and-a-half later, they made their plans again, and this time Terry showed with only enough money for two bus tickets back to North Carolina. Without even enough money to feed my fourteen-year-old sister or herself, Terry asked at the various cafes along the way home if they could spare a free meal because her purse had been stolen and she needed to feed her child. Luckily some gave them free meals and they managed to eat well during their road trip.

Back at home, I was shocked and felt abandoned. I was angry that Sheila hadn't considered the impact of her actions on me before she ran away. She hadn't even told me she was in touch with Terry. How could she do that to me? Did I not mean anything to her?

Sheila rang once shortly after she moved back with Terry to tell me she was in love with a man. I asked her quite seriously what love was, and she explained to me in a way that I would most understand. She said, 'You know when you make two peanut butter and jelly sandwiches, and one of them is better than the other? Well, love is choosing to give the other person the better sandwich because you want them to be happy.' Until not so long ago, I believed that loving a person meant putting their every need before my own to make them happy and prove my devotion, even if it meant I starved.

I didn't talk to Sheila again for two and a half years, and wouldn't see her again for another eight. During that time she was abandoned by Terry again shortly after moving to North Carolina, had her first serious relationship with a man Terry set her up with called 'Crackers,' met a man named Wayne whom she married at age sixteen, and had her first baby, Lora Lee, the same year. A further two daughters quickly followed. I know a lot of partying, sex, drugs, and rock-n-roll lifestyle went on during that time, and that's probably why I didn't hear from Sheila.

Shortly after I learned Sheila was with Terry again, I received a letter from Tina. Separated at the Dependent Unit five years earlier, it was the first time I had heard from her. Age 17, she wrote:

Dear Laura, How you doing babe. I miss you so much. I'm sorry I haven't written you sooner. But I hope your doing good with your new family. I had plans but I guess it was just a dream. Well whatever happy Birthday day and merry x-mas kinda late. (oh Laura I'm sorry and I love you so much). I just want to hold you and tell you so. Well you wouldn't believe what I'm been through. I'm Canadian Texas. I love it here. I got a job I pay my own rent and I don't do dope any more. I go to church now. I guess you could say I've gone straight. The other night I was put in jail, because I had a warrant for running away from California but I talked to Sally and she said I was doing good and could stay. So I'm free really free. I can't believe it. That and you was all I ever wanted. I love you. That's why I feel more for you than Sheila of course I love her to but I still mis-place her for what she did to me. Laura when your old enough to understand you will. Well Laura I really can't wait to hear from you. Will you call me. I can't call you cause I got a phone bill up to my neck. So heres my phone number if you want to call (806-323-8088) well Laura I'm gonna cut this short I don't really feel good spending that night in jail really shook me up so write and please call. I love you very much. Love you very much and Always and Forever. Bye love. Tina Wallace. PS. I met my real dad but he molested me. Kiss Kiss. Kisses to you.'

Attached to my letter was a letter written to my parents in capital letters:

'DEAR MR & MRS BOYNTON, THANK YOU FOR WHAT YOUR DOING FOR HER. AND PLEASE TAKE CARE OF HER. I LOVE HER MORE THAN ANYTHING. I MIGHT NOT SHOW IT RIGHT NOW. BUT I DO WITH ALL MY HEART. SO PLEASE LOVE HER AND SHOW HER THAT YOU DO. SEND A PICTURE OF YOU TOO PLEASE. BUT IF YOU CAN SEND A LOT OF HER SO I CAN PUT THEM IN MY PHOTO ALBUM AND SAVE THEM. AND I WILL KNOW THAT SHE'S HERE WITH ME AND I'LL HAVE SOMETHING TO KEEP NEAR MY HEART LIKE I WAS HOLDING HER MYSELF. THANK YOU AGAIN AND TAKE CARE. LOVE TINA

Tina saw me as her baby because she virtually raised me while Terry was doing what Terry did best – getting drunk and sleeping around. My poor sister was taking on adult responsibilities at such a tender age. She never had a childhood of her own and when she did have an opportunity to be young and carefree, she didn't know how. She was constantly trying to live up to Terry's expectations and earn her love, and felt one way she could do this was by mirroring Terry's behaviour and bad habits. What it actually did was remind Terry of what a bad mother she had been, and what a screwed up woman she was. In Terry's eyes, she hadn't let us down – it was Tina. Tina grew up paying for Terry's mistakes.

About a year after Tina sent me her letter, I received a telephone call from her informing me she was now living back in Healdsburg near Santa Rosa, California with her new husband Allan. She had moved in with Allan the day they met, and together they bought, sold and consumed vast amounts of speed. Of course, when I virtually dropped the phone and ran to see her, I had no idea what sort of life they were leading. She looked great, and it felt like we had never been apart. She was so happy, beautiful and full of life. Her husband was tall and thin with blond hair, and both were very young but appeared smitten with each other. They took me swimming on the Russian River with Allan's sister and we had a wonderful day making up for lost time. When it came time to say goodbye is when all the pain returned. Mom and Dad kept promising me it wouldn't be long before I saw her again, but I had heard that before, so it didn't mean much.

Chapter 20

A moment of rest

In 1981, my new family and I moved to another place in Belmont. I remember the year clearly because it was the year that Prince Charles and Lady Diana Spencer married and the year that I decided I wanted to live in England in one day.

In my new school I made many new friends and enjoyed simple childhood pleasures like playing Hippolyta in the Shakespeare play 'A Midsummer Night's Dream' with a breathtaking assortment of lines which consisted of my only line, 'And then the moon, like a silver bow, shall behold our wedding ceremony.' My teacher was really cross with me because I refused to wear stage makeup saying that my mother doesn't allow me to wear it. He resorted to calling her and asking very politely if she wouldn't mind having words with me. Once I got the go ahead, I happily complied. I just wanted to please.

Although I dressed sweetly in the things Mom had bought or even made for me, nobody ever crossed my path in the wrong way twice. Yes, I was easy going. I even won 'Best Personality' at the end of year awards that were given by students to other students. I was no pushover though and was certainly never bullied. Most of my fellow classmates seemed to recognise that in me, but there was always the odd one that wanted to test my resolve.

Whilst playing tetherball one day during recess (a game played in the States where a volleyball hangs on a chain from a 10 ft stationary metal pole, and two players stand on opposite sides trying to hit the ball one way; one clockwise, and one counter-clockwise), a girl known for being tough queued in my line. When it was her turn to play against me, she walked up and poked me in the chest with her finger and told me I was going to lose this game. True to my inbred fighting nature, I made a split second decision to make it clear who was boss of me. I backed up a step, took the chain and ball, and swung them hard around her arm so that it became locked between the pole and the chain. It must have hurt. In fact, it was meant to. I didn't say anything. I just stood there looking into her eyes with a cold stare while she cried. When I felt I had made my point, I let the chain go, it unwound itself from her arm and the pole, and she ran away. I never went looking for trouble, but when it presented itself, I was too unwise to back down from it.

During this year, Mom took me out of class one day to see a specialist about my back, which was curving in a 'S' shape. After waiting around for hours in a community hospital and subsequent x-rays, I was diagnosed with scoliosis, a severe curvature of the spine that needed correcting with a back brace.

For over a year I had to wear under my clothes the most hideous back brace ever invented. Extending from just under my breasts to the top of my pelvic bone, it made me look half robot and half human. Hard white plastic wrapped around my front to my back, cinching me in and keeping me straight by pulling two large pieces of Velcro at the back. It was the same size and concept as a corset except a lot thicker and harder. It was hard to bend down (God forbid I dropped my pencil), and every time I sucked my tummy in and let it out, it made a farting noise. This, as it happened, came in handy one day when I accidentally farted loudly in class and blamed it on my back brace. I wondered if I would ever just be a 'normal' child with 'normal' problems.

I saw Tina once during this year. When my parents and I arrived on the day Tina and I had agreed on, Tina was stoned and couldn't remember speaking to me or arranging the visit. I stayed with her for the weekend and it became clear to me that not everything was tickety-boo. She and Allan were fighting quite a bit, and it was obvious they were drinking and smoking far too much pot. When my parents came to pick me up, we all went to dinner and Mom and Dad spent the better part of the meal trying to give them couple counselling. Tina was upset that Allan never took her anywhere, like dancing or out for a meal, and that he was always going out on his own. Allan said he needed time and space to himself. They went round and round about possible solutions, but neither seemed satisfied with the answer, and it certainly didn't help that Tina was pregnant with their first child.

Later that summer I had a boyfriend who lived just around the corner from me. He wrote me about 10 notes a day on his astrological space ship stationary, dropped them through my letterbox and ran. I returned the favour – except my stationary had pastel crayons across the bottom. One day he didn't drop any notes through my letterbox and I feared he had abandoned me, so I wrote him a long letter saying so. In return I received a short note back saying, 'I write you everyday, and the only time I don't, I get this!' That was my first realisation that maybe I was a bit too sensitive, and that boys definitely don't think as girls do.

To make up for my inadequacies, I plucked up enough courage to invite him and three girlfriends around for a shaving cream fight in my back yard. Mom and Dad didn't allow boys in the house when they weren't home, but surely the back garden was OK, right? First, we walked to the local Walgreen's and bought several cans of shaving cream. Then we stopped for an ice cream before returning to my house.

We chased each other around my back garden covering each other from head to toe in shaving cream. Although we were having a marvellous time, it soon became clear that we hadn't really thought it through. Once we were finished and my friends had no clean clothes to change into, I had to hose them off. Now drenched, we said goodbye and I watched them squelch down my road and out of sight leaving a path of wet footsteps behind. I held them in my mind's eye for a few minutes after they turned the corner and disappeared. I did this often in my younger years, breathed in the moment and appreciated how wonderful the colours and sounds made me feel. It meant a great deal to have fun, carefree days with great friends like them. For once I felt like I easily fit in and belonged. Never mind that I had turned my back on the past and my feelings. I had pushed thoughts of who I was in the recent past and how I felt about myself deep down, squashing them into a condensed cube of heavy lead that I was burdened to carry with me the rest of my life.

The following day my boyfriend dropped the following note through my door that I have kept all these years:

> *Dear Lora, I hope we can do another fun thing this week. I just got a new watch with alot of gagits that I haven't figured out how to use I'd like to show it to you. I just finist a letter to my dad before you called and I'm pretty sure I'm not going so me and you can do a lot of things this summer. I hope you can come up in my room as soon as I clean it. Then you can see my snake if you are not scared of them. I think the letters you gave me are very cute and so are the stickers. Remember what you said in*

your last note that I looked handsome the last day of
school well you are pretty all the time!

A few days later, sat outside in my back garden, I wanted to write
a poem that summarised how I'd been feeling. I looked around
taking in my environment; the white rabbit hutch with Peaches
in it, the subsequent flies, the plum tree, the picnic table I sat at,
the bees buzzing around the golden marigolds Mom planted
every year, and the cool uplifting breeze most welcome on such
a hot day. I felt dreamy and removed. I had it! I wrote my poem
and bounded into the house with my fist full of paper cheering,
'Mom! I've just written my first poem!' I read it to her proudly:
'See the birds. See the bees. See the flies fly around me.'

'Lora, don't say *see the flies fly around me*. It sounds bad.'

I went away in deep thought and later changed it to 'see the
butterflies fly around me' and was happy again (although
between you and me it really was flies).

Chapter 21

Little 'K' and Elvis

Mom still couldn't conceive a child of her own, so my parents decided to adopt a baby. They learned of a baby that had been conceived when an Irish woman met a Spanish man in a janitor's closet on the psychiatric ward where they were both patients. I know, sounds like the beginning of a bad joke. Unfit and unable to care for a baby, the woman was giving her child up for adoption. When my parents were asked if they were interested in adopting the baby, despite being warned it would most likely have psychological problems and difficulties in the future, they were so desperate for a baby of their own they jumped at the chance.

I was with Mom and Dad's friends skiing in Lake Tahoe, while they stayed back to make sure they were at the hospital when the baby was born. I called a few times a day asking if my new brother or sister had arrived yet only to be told, 'not yet dear.' Finally, on the 13th March, twelve years younger than I, my new little sister Katharine Suzanne arrived.

When I got home a couple of days later, I bounded into the house excited to see my sister. She was dressed in the most beautiful little girl things I had ever seen. She wore white tights and a

95

lovely frilly yellow dress and smelled of sweet baby shampoo and powder. Her hair looked like a little a monkey's – black, long and sticking out as if she had received an electric shock. Mom allowed me to hold her, and although it was a new experience to hold a baby so fragile and young, it was not awkward for me in the least. I immediately bonded with my sweet baby sister.

I enjoyed being the eldest sister for a change. I did things like take her to the park and on bus rides to the local mall to walk around and show her off. At first I called her Katharine, but soon replaced that with 'Little K', and not much later shortened it even further to 'Kay' and it stuck.

Mom said I was jealous of Kay, but I didn't feel jealous. I learned a lot about how to care for babies through watching Mom handle her. I wondered if Terry was ever so affectionate and doting, or did she always leave me to fend for myself? Did I get a beautiful room with lovely stuffed animals, bright colours, a wardrobe stuffed full of new gorgeous girly clothes? Or was I always dressed in second hand clothes and playing with dead rats and cockroaches for entertainment? Did Terry ever tickle and coo at me, sing to and cherish me as Mom did Kay, or was I always frightened, neglected and alone?

I vowed that when I had babies I was going to be the best mother possible. I would give them everything I missed and adore them the way children are meant to be. I would be interested in their lives and would be there when they fell and needed dusting off. I would make them smell yummy with fresh clothes and clean hair, and tell them how much I loved them at all times. You just wait: I would make it different for my children.

Kay followed me around like a puppy. Every time I was eating something, she would toddle over with her mouth open waiting for me to put food into it. Once when I was spraying whip cream onto a bowl of ice cream, she came as she always did and kept saying, 'keem Sissy, keem.' I finally had enough and stuck the nozzle in her mouth and sprayed. Then something overtook me. I filled her mouth and didn't stop. In the end, whip cream was all over her – on her face, out her nose, on her front. We were both laughing hysterically and continued to laugh about it for many years. After that she was more cautious about asking for whatever it was I was eating!

I taught Kay a few of her firsts. She would spend hours with me in my room, so it was no surprise that the first song she learned was, 'All Shook Up', followed by 'Miss Me,' by Culture Club. Another first I taught her was how to drink out of a straw. Both firsts were silly things perhaps, but things that bonded us together none the less.

Meanwhile like many other Americans, I believed I was immune to events of the world. Things would sort themselves out the way they always do. Cocooned in a world of sister-ship, friendship, laughter, Mc Donald's, hot dogs, Coca Cola, Twix's, Guess jeans, Ralph Lauren and the slow discovery of what boys are actually good for, I had no real worries anymore.

It was around this time that I suddenly remembered I loved Elvis Presley. I felt ashamed that I had forgotten him since he had died. One moment I was repeatedly throwing myself off a rock in the middle of the Russian River in demonstration of my grief over his death, and the next I was eating copious amounts of chocolate chip ice cream without a worry in the world. I was a traitor! One night I wrote him a long letter saying how sorry I was, folded it up, and placed it on my shelf before I went to bed. As I fell asleep, I imagined his spirit coming in the night to read it.

I also joined a fan club and dragged my parents and friends to see endless Elvis impersonators at various fairs. At one show the impersonator took his sweaty scarf from around his fat neck and handed it to me in the audience. I thought I had died and gone to heaven.

Through the Elvis fan club, I made a new pen pal from England. Although he was eighteen and I was only twelve, this didn't stop us from writing about how much we loved and were devoted to Elvis. When we weren't sharing our vast knowledge of Elvis facts, my pen pal told me all about England. Over time I developed my fascination about a far away land that would stick with me for years to come.

In my journal I talked about Elvis constantly, writing things like, 'Lora – when you get married I want somebody to sing the Hawaiian wedding song that Elvis sang in Blue Hawaii.' Under the section entitled 'Important Dates' I listed the most important dates I could think of: 'August 2nd – Mom's b-day. August 4th – real Mom's b-day. August 2nd – sister Sheila's b-day. August 16th 1977 – Elvis died! March 13th – sister Kay's b-day. January 8th 1935 – Elvis' b-day. April 20th – Dad's b-day. July – Elvis Now's Fan Club Anniversary. July 4th (Independence Day) – started my period.' On every other page I wrote, 'I love Elvis Presley – he's such a fox.' What amuses me most is how I ended most entries with, 'Elvisly Yours, Lora.' This was the closest I came to acknowledging my past.

Chapter 22

Alice

In 1983, age 13, I started junior high school, and had a handful of new friends, but it was Alice with whom I was closest. We soon discovered we had two huge things in common: we were both in love with Josh Finkelstein and Boy George of Culture Club. I guess we both have a thing for big noses. From the moment we met, we were inseparable. Alice was petite and had short blond hair and brown eyes. Both of us at the time were 'wanna-be preppies' wearing all the right designer clothes. I like to believe that even when we were dressing like everybody else, we had a unique, artistic flair about how we presented ourselves – something just a little different.

Alice was really easy going. She giggled a lot and had a warm and engaging quality. Even though I was a far more serious character than she, one that tended to over think everything, when she laughed she would squint her eyes into crescents and pull her shoulders up towards her cheeks deep in the feel of laughing. I couldn't help but fall about laughing too, letting go of all the drama that plagued me deep inside.

In history class the desks were positioned in a U-shape, and Alice and I sat opposite Josh. Besides Josh's big nose, we also liked that he was a 'preppy' wearing two Ralf Lauren Polo shirts with turned up collars (he liked to layer them), and argyle socks and penny loafers on his feet. We laughed and giggled whilst pointing at him. In embarrassment he covered his face with his woolly jumper. When he brought it down again there was an enormous piece of white fluff on his eyelashes that he kept trying to blink away. That was it. Alice and I literally fell out of our seats laughing and our teacher threatened to separate us if we didn't quieten down.

Sometimes when I spent the night at Alice's house we saw Josh at his friend Charlie's. They would hang out in the driveway just opposite Alice's bedroom window. Both pretended they didn't see us spying down on them; they just happened to like hanging out in driveways, kicking tyres on parked cars without speaking much. Alice and I wrote a song about Josh that went, 'If you're walking down the street and happen to see the nose, the shoes, the socks, the shirt…. Tell Finkel-snoz he can go with the dirt!'

When I asked Alice about her memories of this time, she said:

> *I always felt completely free with you. I was ready for you and me to up and move to London back in '84. Ever since Jr. High, you made me feel happy to be me and not so awkward and insecure. You made me laugh and not care what anyone else thought. And best of all, you saw the 'sexy' in Joshua Finkelstein.*

For one of the first times in my life I wasn't merely surviving; I was genuinely happy and content. I was at a place where I could finally relax and not worry about where my next meal would come from (although Mom says I did continually ask just to make sure.) I didn't climb into my closet to sleep at night, fearful that a stranger may come and take me away. I had no more nightmares about a huge monster gobbling me up, and even my separation from Sheila seemed to have its benefits — like not having to share. I was living in the moment, rolling with gentle day-to-day lapping waves and appreciating every moment.

I even started to think about the future. Because I love animals, I thought I wanted to train as a veterinarian. Although I wasn't sure about having to stick my arm up a cow's bottom like Mom said I'd have to. I also loved the idea of being an archaeologist in a hot desert under make-do tents discovering the world's oldest artefacts. Mom said that I could go years without actually finding anything, so I had to give that some thought too.

The following year, age fourteen, Alice and I started high school. I enjoyed taking French lessons and art, and developed my love for the English language. My English teacher tucked me under his wing and encouraged my interests by offering me a book of poems he had written and kindly commented on the ones I wrote in return. I only remember him saying he liked one, which went something along the lines of, 'Friends are like a fine crystal glass. You must treat them with care. Hold them up and appreciate their beauty. For if you mishandle them, they may shatter, and you'll never be able to put the pieces back together again.' That was the gist of it. Although, I'd like to think it sounded a bit better than the tale of Humpty Dumpty fell off the wall...

One evening Alice and I went into Millers Outpost retailers. There we saw a Look Alike Nick Rhodes (member of the '80's band Duran Duran), whom we happened to adore. He even had the same dyed blond fringe. We were in love. We hung out amongst the clothes eyeing him until closing time when we helped him tidy the clothes and got to chat. He finally pushed us out so he could pull down the gates and go home, and we exchanged telephone numbers full of excitement.

As we always did everything in pairs, the following week we both rang Look Alike Nick and asked if he'd like to go out to dinner with us, and, oh yeah, my family too. Surprisingly, he agreed. We met him at the Iron Gate Restaurant on El Camino Real. My parents sat at one table, and Alice, Look Alike Nick and I sat around another. During dinner, middle names came up and Look Alike Nick and I couldn't believe we both had the same middle name Lee. I asked Alice what her middle name was, and when she responded, 'Virginia,' I spat out my drink in a fit of laughter. I don't know why, but both Look Alike Nick and I couldn't contain ourselves, leaving Alice rather annoyed.

A couple of days later, Look Alike Nick rang and asked me out on a date. Mom said I could go on one condition: I had to tell him I was only 15 years old. If he still wanted to see me after that, it was OK to go. During a telephone conversation, I said to him very nervously, 'Isn't it funny how you just turned 19 and I'm only 15?' Met with a punishing silence on the other end of the line, he eventually flatly replied, 'Oh.' Once he overcame his shock, he dated me anyways. He was my first serious boyfriend in that we actually kissed, cuddled and did other things couples do – except one.

I told Mom and Dad I was spending the night at Alice's house, which was a risky strategy because I hadn't told Alice I used her as an alibi. If she had known, she would have been very cross with me because when she is put under fire she can't tell a lie if her life counted on it. The gamble paid off, and instead of spending the night with my friend, I was checking into the *Bel-Mateo* motel on El Camino Real with Look Alike Nick. We had reached that point in our relationship where we wanted to do the one thing that we hadn't yet done... that neither of us had ever done. He switched on the TV and went into the bathroom for an extraordinarily long time. He started running the shower as I stretched out on the bed wondering if he was having a wash before we did the dirty deed. Eventually he came out fully clothed and explained that he had to have a 'dump' and hadn't wanted to smell up the room. Nice touch. I guess it could have been worse; we could have been doing it in the back of his station wagon.

The next morning as I climbed out of Look Alike Nick's 'Woody' station wagon on the way to breakfast, I experienced a severe pain in my right leg just below my knee causing me to nearly collapse. I thought it was a pulled muscle from running track at school, so I rented crutches to get around on and thought nothing more of it.

Within a week, the pain in my leg had subsided but a large lump had formed where the pain had once been. My parents took me to see a specialist who recommended a biopsy to rule out the 'C' word. On the day, as I was wheeled into surgery, I was strongly assured that it was 'probably just a calcium build up.'

Just before I awoke from the general anaesthetic, I had a dream where I said through hysterical tears, 'Just a calcium build up, huh?' In reality, I bolted upright in my hospital bed and stared at the clock that read 5:14 pm. It was already dark outside – the days are short this time of year. Once the nurses brought me back to my room, I stared out the windows into blackness still feeling sleepy from the anaesthetic. Suddenly a handful of my closest friends gushed through the door to my side. They were crying, and one blurted out through sobs, 'You only have a 10% chance of surviving!' This was before my parents had even had a chance to tell me the bad news; it was cancer.

I will only ever have one youth. It had just ended. It was floating away steadily like a helium balloon. There was no way it was coming back, and all I could do was watch the last chance of any normality climb higher and higher until just a speck consumed by nothingness. I have never been content to let anything end in anti-climax, and I didn't disappoint. Shocked, numb and feeling emotionally exposed, I retreated deep into myself once again, staring blankly at my four inner walls that over the years had become my cell. I felt as if it wasn't me anymore, I was a shadow of myself looking down, already dead and in another place.

Loneliness: the word that keeps visiting me like a lover in the night filling me with desire and longing but never fulfilling its promise; the word that holds my heart tightly in its fist and is capable of squeezing all life from me. How could I possibly fit in or be happy now? I would never be normal or have it easy no matter how hard I tried.

There weren't many times after Terry left when I really missed her, but this was one of the rare instances when I ached for her, my mommy – the person who should have been there making everything better with a hug. I rocked back and forth like a baby, holding my arms around myself crying repeatedly, 'Mommy' with every ounce of desire in me. The worst part was the realisation that I had been robbed of the 'mommy' that I was crying for. My soul ached for her but I knew she was just a fantasy.

Sheila rang once after my diagnosis and told me she would name her first born, due any day, after me. She said Terry knew I was ill, but never once did Terry make the effort to ring and see how I was coping with treatment. That was all the proof I needed that I was right; 'Mommy' was just a figment of my imagination.

For a few days following my diagnosis, my friends and Look Alike Nick hung out in my room after school, joking around about who would get what when I died. One friend said she definitely had to have my electric nail polish dyer. It was all said tongue in cheek, and I think had any one of us really comprehended how serious the situation was, distasteful jokes like that would hurt. As it was, the reality hadn't sunk in for any of us, and we were just being the silly teenagers we had always been.

A week later, my parents and I arrived at the Paediatric Department of Kaiser Permanente for my first meeting with Dr Patrick Hardy, the doctor who would prescribe my chemotherapy treatment. A big boned, broad-chested, large bellied, short man with short curly greying hair sat behind a desk in a boring beige hospital office. Like naughty school children, my parents and I sat at the front of his desk wearing our best clothes and behaviour.

He looked straight into my eyes with a hardened cold stare I didn't anticipate or deserve and said, 'You have cancer. You may die. If you're not going to take this seriously – don't waste my time.' I thought, *I hate you! I didn't ask to have this, so don't blame me if I feel angry about it*, and that was the beginning of our doctor/patient relationship.

As if having cancer wasn't bad enough, before treatment started Look Alike Nick said he had something of great importance he needed to tell me. We sat in his car one night parked outside my parent's house and my hard drilling began; he was going to make me work very hard for whatever it was he needed to tell me. He kept saying it was very bad – very dirty. The windows were fogging up, and my curfew was eminent. He drew on the front steamed up window a 'G' and said it began with that. He then lay across my lap as I stroked his forehead asking him what could possibly be so bad. He finally said, 'I think I'm a little...' and wagged his hand in a gesture that at first looked like it was miming the word 'no.' Then it sunk in that his pinkie and forefinger were sticking out. *Oh my God...*

'Are you Gay?' I asked with exclamation in my voice rather than question.

He nodded yes in a little girl fashion, blinking his long eyelashes up at me.

I pushed him onto the floor of his car and got out, slamming the door. He didn't follow. As I walked like a zombie towards my front door, I thought, *is my life some sort of sick joke? Can this really be happening to me?*' I opened the front door; Mom took one look at me, saw my *Oh my God* expression and said, 'he's gay' not with question in her voice, but with absolute certainty. How did she know? Was I the only person on earth who couldn't see it?

I felt like there was an invisible giant cat and I was the little mouse that was played with and knocked around from side to side. When the cat lost interest from time to time, I scrambled to get away and just when I thought it was safe, its paw returned and batted me around some more. I wondered when it would finally get tired with its game and put me out of my misery.

Not long after, Look Alike Nick moved to Los Angeles with the boy who he claimed he loved, leaving me to fight two evils at once – cancer and abandonment. Not just abandoned by my gay ex-boyfriend, but most of my friends suddenly disappeared too. The only friend that remained true and constant was Alice, and because she was the only friend left, I relied on her heavily for the next year and more.

Following my diagnosis and learning that Look Alike Nick was gay, late one night I sat on my futon in my room in deep emotional pain. Tired of feeling like a parcel that had no control over its destination, I decided if anything would end my life, it would be me. It was the only sense of control I could find. I held the large bottle of codeine tablets given to me following my biopsy, opened the lid and filled my fist full. I sat for over an hour in deep thought trying to decide if I really wanted to end my life.

I made my decision; I slowly and methodically drank down each tablet and laid down, fully expecting to never wake again.

In the night I woke up swollen, covered head to toe in hives and feeling very, very ill. In violent spasms, my stomach rejected everything in it. To this day, I still can't take codeine without being sick.

The next day Tina came from Healdsburg to visit. I hadn't told her what I had attempted the night before, and once I saw my sister I felt ashamed for trying to end my life without having even considered her. She took Alice and me to the mall in her baby blue Ford pick up truck, and on the way home honked the horn at some good looking guys that were walking along El Camino Real. We laughed loudly out the windows when the guys nearly jumped out of their skin. The roles had reversed and now they knew how it felt!

Later that evening, Tina and I stayed up late and watched Prince's movie, *Purple Rain*. We laughed a lot and I wondered why on earth less than twenty-four hours before I had been so depressed I had wanted to end my life. The next day Tina left, but the happiness I felt with her around did not. Within me there was a renewed sense of fight.

Chapter 23

Treatment

My doctor and parents kept telling me how horrible treatment would be and to prepare myself for what was coming, but I thought – *No! I'll show them how tough I am. They'll see that with the right mindset it won't be nearly as difficult as they make out.*

I arranged for a friend to meet me at the hospital to keep me company during my first treatment, then put on my fake eyelashes as I always did, drew on my thick Boy George makeup, dressed in my punk clothes and headed off for the hospital with Dad. On arrival, in my own private room I changed into my hospital gown and talked with the nurse cheerfully as she looked for a vein to administer the medicine.

'You're awfully cheerful today Lora Lee' said the nurse.

'Yep! Why shouldn't I be?'

'Huh' she said unconvinced.

She easily found a vein, connected the intravenous drip and left the room. Twenty minutes later I was begging between retches for the nausea to stop. As I filled a bucket with the contents of my stomach, I felt my fake eyelashes leak down my cheeks in tears. My friend never showed and Dad said he stayed with me the whole day and into the night before driving me home, but I don't remember him being there. All I remember is throwing up for over eight hours and then Dad driving me home while I threw up in a bucket in the car. He says I was so concentrated on being ill that everything else didn't seem to exist.

I never admitted that not only was the treatment as bad as they had said it would be – it was a million times worse.

A week or so after my first chemotherapy session, I was sitting on Alice's loo running my fingers through my hair. Alarmingly, large clumps simply fell out and filled my hands. In shock, I couldn't stop running my hands through just to see how much more would come. Without resistance, my hair kept filling handful after handful. I wasn't prepared for that. In fact, I freaked out. I jumped off the loo, pulled up my pants and trousers, and ran to Alice in hysterical tears.

Like most things, Alice was good about it, taking it in her stride as if she had seen this a hundred times before. Her strong maternal instincts and deep rooted need to help took over; before I knew what was happening we were at Walgreen's Pharmacy buying some funky hair dye to colour my remaining hair bright red. Alice then styled my hair into a Mohawk for a couple of weeks, but eventually the remaining hair was so thin, she helped me shave that off too. She was always so great like that. She was one of the only people I felt comfortable enough to take my wig off in front of, and when I did, she'd do things like draw swastikas on my head to make me look and feel more punk than ill. She told me I was lucky – that she had always wanted to shave her head, but her parents wouldn't let her. No doubt she would have looked better than I did with my huge Dumbo ears.

The wigs I chose to wear were never very serious. I didn't try to pretend that I wasn't wearing one. In fact, I went the opposite direction and bought the most outlandish, funky and fun wigs I could find. Mom nearly died when I took the expensive, real longhaired wig she bought me and cut it down to a short punky style and died it jet-black. I needed to personalise it. I may have had cancer, but cancer didn't have me.

Alice wrote me an email about her memory of that time:

> *The thing I remember about you losing your hair was you waking up in the mornings and huge clumps would be left on your pillow. I remember you being heart broken about it and I thought 'well now you can just shave your head like I always wanted to do'. But you really held on to it as long as you could. It was a good thing you had such a great sense of style. I remember the hat with the ponytail that we taped to the top of your head so you could have bangs. Also, the real hair wig that cost so much money, but you hated it, so you cut it and dyed it black. I don't think your mom was very happy. But my favourite was the blond wig. Thank god it was the 80's because cancer and all, you didn't skip a beat 'fashion wise'.*

Unfortunately there are some cruel people out there, particularly amongst my peers at school. I will never forget the embarrassment of people staring and pointing at me as I walked down the school's corridor. I went from being looked at because I was attractive to being gawked at because I was now considered a freak. Those who had once spoken to me because they liked me now spoke to me as if I had a disease they could catch. Some spoke sickly sweet words delivered in a holier than thou manner, while suddenly others who I didn't even know wanted to be my friend because I was now considered a cause that could help them feel they were contributing to the world.

Then there was the time a young man who attended my high school asked me out on a blind date. I went along curious who he may be. On the way to the restaurant he popped a tape in and hit PLAY. A song with the lyrics, 'when you think of Laura, laugh – don't cry, I know she'd want it that way...' filled my ears with horror as he explained he always thought of me when he played that song. I should have asked him to take me home right then because for the rest of the date I didn't hear a word he said. I was filled with rage at the possibility he felt he could have me because I was ill. Just because I had cancer didn't mean I would lower my standards. I don't know why I felt that way. I felt many irrational things at the time. He was probably a very nice guy who felt he was being charitable, but I didn't want charity. I wanted everybody to treat me as I was used to – like me.

By my third treatment it dawned on me that I wasn't going to be given a gold medal for having a positive attitude, which didn't seem to help matters anyway. I became so frightened of treatment that just smelling rubbing alcohol made me sick. My doctor could no longer easily find veins and my once cheerful attitude was replaced with attitude full stop. When my doctor missed yet another vein I decided to make my feelings known and tell him exactly what I was thinking. 'Owwww!' I growled. 'That fucking hurts you know! Asshole.' I said while he hunted down another vein.

Dr Hardy laughed, which made me angrier.

'Do you get some sort of sick joy out of nearly poisoning me to death?' I asked with snake eyes.

"Yeah. It's the first thing I think of when I wake up in the morning; *gee, who can I poison today? I know, let's poison Lora Lee'* he replied sarcastically.

I couldn't help but say 'Jerk' with half a smile.

'I do what I have to.'

Throughout my gruelling chemotherapy treatment, which lasted 50 weeks and involved taking Cytoxin pills every day for 7 days then an intervenes drip of Adriamycin on the 8th day, my attitude deteriorated from bad to worse. It was very intensive to have chemotherapy every couple of weeks for over a year; the thought alone would frighten and weaken the strongest of people. I was no different. There were no drugs to help with nausea. I knew exactly what was about to happen and would panic. I didn't want to be puking the inside lining of my stomach up for hours – to the point where I didn't even know where I was, or what day it was.

Subsequently I started running away before each treatment. Sometimes I'd go and stay with a friend whose mother was single and worked full time. We had the house to ourselves all day, and at night I hid in her closet until her mother went to bed. One day we had a load of our gay friends over and they grabbed me, pinned me down on the bed and proceeded to drip hot wax from a burning candle onto my bare stomach. It was all done in good spirits, but what bothers me most now is when I think, *What if? What if they hadn't been just a bunch of gay guys being silly with their good friend? What if they were straight guys, then what may have happened?* I cringe now at all the times I was so vulnerable and didn't even realise it. As it was, it turned out to be their way of foreplay and before long the room turned into one large orgy. My girlfriend and I went into the other room and watched TV.

I stayed with my friend for a couple of weeks before the police picked me up in Kentucky Fried Chicken one evening. I was taken home and subsequently forced to have my treatment. This process soon became the norm; every couple of weeks I would run away, stay with various friends and would eventually be found by the police and forced to have treatment.

When my parents started locking me in my room at night so I couldn't run away before treatment, I adopted new tactics. I would pack a light bag, open my window, take my folded futon and squeeze it through my second storey bedroom window, and let it drop to the ground. I carefully climbed out the window and hung from the window frame before letting go, hoping I landed on the futon. How I managed to do it without breaking a leg is a mystery. Once out my window I would leave by the side gate and walk to El Camino Real and catch a bus towards one of my friends' houses.

On another occasion, I stayed in a two-bedroom apartment with at least ten other clubbers and punks. All they did every day, besides smoke cigarettes and dope, was lay in a heap on a bed watching *The Price is Right* and *Spin the Wheel*. The place was clearly overcrowded but I was allowed to stay on the condition I cleaned up after everybody. What a nightmare, the place was a dump. There were no distinguishable piles of clothes and dishes – it was one big mess. It was better than treatment though, so I happily got stuck in. Then one day the guy whose name was on the lease told me I had to leave because when he had agreed to let me stay he didn't realise I was wanted by the police. I was too dangerous for them because too many of them were wanted.

Once, a day before a treatment, a group of friends came to my front door to collect me. Dad knew what this meant – that I wouldn't be coming home that night and the chase would be on. He appealed to my friends, 'Please don't take her. Leave her here. She needs treatment. If she doesn't have treatment she will die. Do you understand? SHE WILL DIE' he pleaded. They didn't say anything and I pushed past Dad to the waiting car. Dad stood on the doorstep with a sad look on his face as we drove away. My gay best friend said, 'YOU'RE GOING TO DIE!' in an exaggerated tone ending it with a Vincent Price laugh. It was the first time I realised that these people I called my friends couldn't care less what happened to me.

When I ran out of people to stay with, my gay best friend (who was also adopted) and I pan handled, and sometimes on my own I would approach taxi drivers at night because I knew they had a wad of cash. I would try to give the impression I was a poor helpless female, and they would give me a couple of dollars. Little did I realise I really was a poor helpless female. A couple of times, I rang the bell at motels and when the owners answered their window in their nightgowns, I explained I had nowhere to sleep. Of course they wouldn't let me have a room, so I asked if they would at least spare a couple of dollars, which they did. When we had enough money for a cup of coffee and some fries, we went to Denny's restaurant and sat there all night drinking coffee refills because we had no other place to go. During the day we went to the park and slept on the grass in the shade.

For meals, I am ashamed to admit that we would eat and run. I didn't like being dishonest, but I was hungry. At one point, I was arrested for trying to steal new underwear and make-up, and even though I was going to such extremes to exist, it never once crossed my mind how dangerous a position I was in as a young woman.

Reading my doctor's assessments of me and how treatment was progressing is quite amusing in hindsight; most patients never have the opportunity. I could hear Dr Hardy's distaste of me through his words:

Lora finally surfaced after her latest run away from home in late February (now April 10th). She completed her final course of chemotherapy consisting of week 50 Cyclophoshamide and Adriamycin and full dosage on March 5th, 1986. Therapy had been delayed three weeks from the protocol schedule due to her disappearance...' and at the end of the letter he says, *'Thank you very much for assisting in this most challenging case. Hopefully Lara's (yes, miss-spelled my name) social problems will be resolved so she can continue to enjoy a favourable outcome.*

Again, another letter written by Dr Hardy:

> *Laura (yes, miss-spelled my name again) has had numerous social difficulties in the past, which are pertinent to her present illness. She is an adopted child, this home since age 8 (I was actually 9). However, there has been a great deal of turmoil with her adjustment to adolescence in recent months, increased during her treatment for Ewing's Sarcoma. She was recently incarcerated at Juvenile Hall for a shoplifting attempt, and has run away from home on these two occasions in recent weeks. Although she states she has complied with oral chemotherapy, it is of question as to how much actual Cytoxan therapy has been taken by the patient since it has not all been supervised by adults. She spent 3 weeks in Hillcrest Juvenile Centre, but is now back in her home although she is currently a ward of the court. She also admits to being regularly sexually active but requests this not be reported to her parents.*

Towards the middle of treatment I met a young man three years older than me. He reminded me of Look Alike Nick, for whom my heart was still bleeding, so I started dating him. In a word, he was too nice, so I'll call him Mr Too Nice. As his name implies, he threw himself at my feet like a red carpet, and being needy, I chose the easy route and walked all over him. In hindsight, I feel incredibly ugly when I consider how I treated him. He was so kind to me, and because I had no self-respect, I thought anybody who could love me the way I was – was obviously a weirdo who didn't deserve my respect. I was so wrong, and I can still hear Mr Too Nice's pain in a comment he posted to me recently:

> *I have to say that I was with you for two of your visits of Chemotherapy at Kaiser in South San Francisco, once Alice joined us in my 68' VW. I was also there the time*

where you pulled the IV out of your arm; it freaked me out because you were in so much pain and there wasn't anything that I could do. I remember running and getting the doctor who told me that, 'Most people would rather be shot by a gun then go through Chemotherapy.' That is when it woke me up to how much pain you were going through. There was a lot leading up to your last treatment that might not make for good reading, but would certainly paint your foster parents in a negative light. I can only say that I don't blame them for all of their behaviour back then, but getting you home a few minutes late after the Til Tuesday concert at Wolfgangs, which led for you to spend days in Juvenile Hall, was certainly uncalled for! After that incident, that is when I decided to help you run away by driving you to Healdsburg some eighty miles away.

After not hearing from you for a week or two I finally decided to tell your step mom of your where abouts; she told me that you had been picked up the night before and I was finally relieved. I remember driving you and Alice back up to Healdsburg for your things and you had broken up with me weeks earlier on the phone because you had cheated on me and were now with JP. (For the record, JP was actually Alice's boyfriend. The boy I cheated on him with was Jaime). *I remember you arriving and going into some house and not coming out for an hour or so, you laughed and asked me what I thought of you? I told you then that I had never said this word to a woman before, but I called you a bitch to your face. I remember that you and Alice laughed and I drove you two back to Belmont; it was miserable. I remember turning down the money your step mom was to give me, and I think you used the money to buy pot; so once again I was contributing to the delinquency of a minor.*

I don't know if this will be posted for all to see, it's not my idea of downplaying anything that you have written, for as close as I could have been with you then you were already pushing me away; so my words really don't matter. These are your memories, not mine.

In retrospect, I feel a great deal of guilt about the way I coped with treatment. Especially when I recall another young girl named Erica who was also receiving treatment at the same time and place for Leukaemia. She was always so well behaved, friendly, patient. Even cheerful! She didn't survive her cancer. I was rotten to my doctor, my family and my boyfriend. I said things I shouldn't have, threw fits, didn't take my Cytoxin pills — yes, his suspicions were justified — ran away from home, stole underwear and food to survive, and I still survived my cancer.

Ultimately I was forced to quit high school because of my medical regime, run away attempts and more honestly because I no longer fitted in. My parents tried home-schooling me, but my tutor was a weak woman and I didn't respect her, so it didn't work out and my education was put on hold.

Instead of going to school, I spent my time going to the mall and hanging out dressed like a mannequin with a long silvery white wig and a heavily painted white face. My reasoning was if people were going to look at me like a freak, I might as well act like one. I played this game where I sat totally still at the base of a statue inside the mall. People walking by stopped and stared; they whispered to each other, 'Is she real?' I got a kick out of it, and it proved to be valuable in connecting me with other outcasts who looked like me. Soon I met a whole gang of teenage misfits, and we loitered all day most days.

In the evenings, my new friends and I went clubbing in San Francisco. Dancing made me feel alive and gave me an outlet for expression. Not only that, but the club scene accepted me just the way I was. In fact, I became like a mini celebrity. Everybody knew me, and I was always given an invite that let me into the clubs for free. For a while, the people I hung out with became my family, looking after me when I'd had too much to drink, making sure I got home or somewhere safe at the end of the night.

More than anything I simply sought the companionship of other young people. I needed desperately to fit in and be a part of a group, to giggle with them and to have what had been missing most of my life: fun and no responsibilities.

It was with this group of friends that I got into quite a lot of trouble. I started smoking cigarettes and marijuana, drinking and occasionally experimenting with other recreational drugs like LSD and XTC. Luckily, this didn't last long. I soon discovered that I didn't actually like altering my reality – it was confusing enough without psychedelic effects. Sometimes when my friends 'dropped acid', I would slip the tab into my pocket and tell them I had taken it so that when they were 'tripping out' I was on parental duty making sure nobody did anything stupid to harm themselves or others. It gave me the opportunity to see how ridiculous a person behaves whilst under the influence of drugs.

Chapter 24

Living with Tina

My exhausted parents needed a break from the drama for a while and asked Tina and Allan if they wouldn't mind having me. I moved into their three-year-old daughter's bedroom, and she moved into Tina and Allan's bedroom to make space. Again, I feel a great deal of guilt because I didn't even appreciate this grand gesture at the time. Of course they made way – of course they cared… I was sixteen and thought the whole universe revolved around me.

I lived with Tina and Allan for about six months. Tina enrolled me into the local high school, and I started a mini version of a new life in Healdsburg.

At first, I settled in.

One day, my teacher asked all his students to come to the front of the class and say what they saw themselves doing or being in the future. When it was my turn I said quite honestly that I saw myself like a character in a soap opera. I imagined that whatever I did and whatever I became would be dramatic and accompanied by exaggerated music for effect. Everybody else talked in terms of a simple life, but I knew even then I wasn't one for blurry memories and nondescript days that would become months and eventually years.

On another day in science, I had a poignant moment as I considered a skeleton hanging in the corner of the classroom. It had been a real person, and I was trying to imagine who the person was that wanted to end up in a classroom full of insolent teenagers who couldn't give a damn. Did the person understand when they donated their body to science that this might be the result?

This started me thinking about how I would like to be handled when I die. The idea of donating my body to science sounded very noble, but did I want to end up hanging in a corner of a classroom rattled and the source of many bad jokes? I thought not. Then I thought of cremation. I had seen a program on TV where they filmed cremation and what happens to a body in the process. Roasting like a chicken didn't do much for me either, thank you very much. I wondered if it smelled as nice, though. Then I thought of the same program where they explained what happens when somebody is prepared for a burial. It's not as innocent as it looks. To preserve the body long enough to last for the funeral, they drain the body's fluids and replace them with formaldehyde. The undertakers paint the body so it looks natural because obviously by now it looks anything but natural. I concluded I didn't want to die at all – none of the options were very nice.

Before long, I had fallen into a bad crowd again. I met my new friends one day as I walked along the street that led from Tina's house to the local 7 – 11 convenience store. I saw a group of outcasts on the opposite side of the road. All of them were punk and unique in their own way, hanging out on the steps of an old Victorian house not doing much of anything, almost as if they were just waiting for me to come along. On the way back from the store, I strategically switched sides of the road. When I approached them, I asked them if they had a cigarette. Conversation ensued and on my very first outing I had made a new pack of friends.

A couple of days later I invited a few of my new friends to Tina's house. The first thing they said was, 'Oh my God, what a total partier's house! Awesome.' I'm not sure what made it look that way the most; maybe it was the 'bong' used for smoking pot that was left on the coffee table, or the distinct lack of decorations and furnishings. Perhaps it was the large TV and closed curtains, or the old, longhaired male lodger sitting on the couch like a zombie. I couldn't quite put my finger on it, but they were right – the place looked similar to Terry's places, which is strange because the house itself was in a new development, and from the outside looked like all the other lovely houses in the cul-de-sac.

Sometimes in the evenings, Tina, Allan, and I would play cards. They would allow me to smoke joints with them, but didn't allow me to drink alcohol. I think their logic was that I had cancer and marijuana had the benefit of helping patients control their nausea. Of course, it was supposed to be smoked during treatment only, but I wasn't arguing.

Tina was around three months pregnant with her second child, so when Allan did a line of cocaine and Tina wanted some, a huge argument would follow resulting in him picking Tina up and placing her outside the front door and locking it. He insisted she couldn't come back in until she had calmed down. I didn't agree with Tina smoking pot, drinking and snorting cocaine whilst she was pregnant, but I also thought it was as equally unfair for Allan to sit there doing all of the above in front of her and then tell her she couldn't have any. It seemed ridiculous in such a dysfunctional situation to begin suggesting that he should support her by not partaking in drugs either.

Tina took me to my second to last chemotherapy treatment. It was a two-hour drive to the hospital and back again, but being the devoted sister, she did it without complaining. Once we were in my private hospital room, before treatment began, Tina asked Dr Hardy if she could smoke a joint with me to help with nausea. To my surprise, he agreed, pulling the curtain around my bed, opening the window, and firmly shutting the door behind him. It was the first time I had smoked marijuana during treatment, and much to my delight it delayed my nausea for several hours.

Once we were home, I went to bed. In the middle of the night, I got up to be sick, and a very hyper and drugged Allan was hopping up and down mad wondering why I was up so late. He was so wired on cocaine, he couldn't even tell how ill I was. Each time I got out of bed to throw up, I had to explain the same thing.

Towards the end of my stay with Tina and Allan, they moved to another older house that looked much more like what Terry used to live in from the inside and out. This time we all had our own rooms. I was supposed to still be taking my Cytoxin pills everyday, but was actually shoving them inside the cover of a large zipped pillow. I didn't see the harm in this at the time. I simply thought I would flush them when nobody was looking.

I don't know why, probably just because I felt like it, I ran away from Tina's and stayed at the same Victorian house where I met my new set of friends. Whilst on the run, my niece unzipped the pillow where I had hidden my Cytoxin pills, and ate some of them. It wasn't until the police picked me up a couple of weeks later that I found out what had happened. Luckily no harm came to my niece but I felt terrible. It was one of the first times I realised what a stupid and horrible thing I had done, and prayed my sister and Allan would forgive me one day for my stupidity.

Meanwhile, now in police custody, I was transferred to Hillcrest

Juvenile Hall in Belmont. Obviously fearing I would run away as soon as I had the chance, the court restrained me long enough to make sure I had my last chemo treatment before my parents agreed to allow me to come home.

On the day of my last treatment I was taken handcuffed to the hospital by a police officer. Before treatment, we stopped at the pathology department so I could leave a urine sample. In the loo, and free from handcuffs, I looked up at the ceiling and clocked the square panels. Desperate to escape while I could, I stood on the toilet seat and tried to reach a panel to see if it would budge. I had the crazy idea that if I could climb into the roof space, I'd drop down somewhere else in the hospital and run to freedom. Despite my best efforts, I couldn't reach and accepted this wouldn't be the place I would make my grand get away.

As soon as I opened the door, the cold heavy handcuffs were replaced. I saw an elderly woman watching. I knew I looked like a criminal sporting jeans and a light blue shirt with 'Hillcrest Juvenile Hall' stamped on the front and back, but I didn't care. As we passed, I smiled at her accusing face and contemplated saying, 'boo!' but didn't want to give her a heart attack. Once in my private room, I was allowed to change into a hospital gown and then sat Indian style on the bed. I distracted myself from what was about to happen by trying to wriggle my wrists free. While I waited anxiously for my doctor, I could hear the police officer's radio crackle in the corridor reminding me he was there. It seemed a bit heavy handed considering I was just a sick sixteen-year-old girl and not a criminal.

'Well hello Lora Lee,' said Dr Hardy as he walked into my private room looking at me in his usual no-bullshit kind of way. 'I see you've finally surfaced from your latest run away attempt,' he said sarcastically as he picked up and read the notes at the foot of my bed.

I jeered at him. We never got along from day one, and that feeling had only intensified throughout my treatment. Surely he could understand why I ran away. Most people would cower at the thought of what he was putting me through. How could he blame me?

Both Dr Hardy and a nurse worked hard to find a vein, but my veins were too clever for them now and immediately disappeared at the faintest smell of rubbing alcohol — a sure sign they were about to be assaulted. As they repeatedly tried to hit a vein, my heart quickened and my hands began to shake and sweat. My stomach cramped and threatened to violently eject everything I had eaten. Like an animal whose life has been threatened, I made a split second decision to scramble to my feet and run for the door. The waiting police officer blocked my way. I didn't know where I was going in my hospital gown and handcuffs, I just knew I had to get out of there. Even though it was my last treatment, my brain simply refused. In a state of panic, I pleaded with them, 'It's my body. It's my choice if I want to die! I hate you. Let….me….GO!' I said as I fought to get past the officer. Realising I would never get past, something in me snapped. I turned around and hysterically clawed at the curtain hanging around my bed pulling it to the floor. The police officer lifted me like a sac of potatoes while I kicked and sobbed, 'No! Put me down.' He plonked me firmly on the hospital bed holding me there until I calmed.

Defeated, my sobs dwindled into whimpers as Dr Hardy began the task of finding a vein again. My hands and arms were covered in purple bruises before he finally found a vein in my foot. He hooked up the intravenous drip and I watched the poison snake its way slowly towards me through a thin tube. The process had begun. Positive I could no longer run away, the police officer removed the handcuffs. I watched with an accusing stare that said *I blame you.*

I had been through treatment countless times and each time the experience was worse than the time before. I knew that in approximately twenty minutes I would be vomiting uncontrollably for hours. I felt like I was stuck on a train track knowing the train was due any minute; I couldn't get away and I knew I was about to be flattened and dragged for miles.

The nausea struck me fast and hard. I quickly lurched forward onto my hands and knees over a bucket on the bed and heaved my breakfast into it. Four hours later I was still retching in rhythmic bursts but only bile was coming. I was exhausted but couldn't stop. Tears and fatigue blurred my vision. My throat burned and the muscles in my stomach cramped in constant pain. There was no longer a world outside my room; it was now just my bucket and me.

Hours later, I was too tired to use my bucket. Lying on my side, I continued to heave. I was too exhausted to even cry. A nurse came into the room and hooked up another bag of saline to keep me hydrated. She said something but I didn't hear her and was too weak to speak. My body was on the brink of death.

Dad picked me up an hour later and brought me home. My heaving had stopped but the nausea persisted. I went straight up to my room and climbed into my welcoming bed. As I felt my spent body sink into the mattress I thought, *Thank God that's it. It's over. I never have to go through that again* and fell into a deep sleep.

Chapter 25

After treatment finished

Treatment had finished and I had beaten the cancer, but the cancer had done its damage. My life didn't stretch before my eyes. My life was right here, right now. No prisoners taken and no apologies made. I never once went back for scans or check-ups. I refused because if I did have cancer again there was no way in hell I would have treatment again. I would have rather died. I was now living for the day – not the future, not looking ahead or feeling any sense of responsibility. I was a 'Wild Child,' as Mom liked to call me.

Somehow, almost miraculously, in between partying and living for the day, I had enough sense to get my GED (General Education Diploma), passing on my first attempt. It is the equivalent to a high school diploma and meant I was in a position to further educate myself in the future, and more importantly to secure basic employment.

Alice had been away for the summer living with her father in Oregon, but she did return towards the end of my treatment. At the time, I felt wounded that she had left me to go and have fun, and being Alice she totally focussed all her attention on her situation at hand – which at the time was her life and friends in Oregon. I wrote in my journal:

I wish she would just stay there the whole summer. It would be a lot better for both of us. We really don't care about each other anymore. At least, I don't and it's evident she doesn't.

Of course I can now clearly see my pain and hurt, and appreciate I was once again trying to cover up my insecurities by being tough. Now that I am older, more sensible and less selfish, I am glad she went away. Just because my childhood had ended, didn't mean hers had to. It must have been a very harrowing experience for her to go through cancer with her best friend. She could have lost me, the one whom she had shared everything. Her mother did the right thing in sending her away from the situation for a while.

When Alice returned from Oregon we resumed where we had left off, except she was depressed and secluded herself more. She no longer talked to me about her feelings, and when I asked her why, she told me it was because she felt she needed to be strong for me. I felt she was pushing me away.

Another thing that changed was instead of staying in, listening to music, talking about boys and writing poetry, we partied and went clubbing in San Francisco. The people we met were such wonderful, colourful people — gay, flamboyant, and fun to hang around. I started to believe I was a 'gay magnet,' as two more boys I dated told me they were gay. It seems obvious with hindsight why I gravitated towards gay men, and why they may have towards me; we were both safe for each other. They weren't the typical men I was used to and certainly didn't want anything from me, and I accepted them for who they were and placed no demands on them. In the end, we did love each other in a plutonic, sisterly kind of way.

With all the changes, when Alice was around she was loyal and supported me through my tribulations. She even went back with me several times to Healdsburg, making my new group of friends hers as well. One time we took a coach from San Francisco up to Santa Rosa to visit Tina because Terry was staying with her, and I wanted Alice to meet my biological mother. At least, that's what I told myself and everybody else, but really I wanted to see Terry. Since she left me at the DU centre I had a few questions that needed answering. Mom and Dad never said how they felt about me going to see Terry, and I never asked. It was just something I had to do.

Tina and Terry picked up Alice and me from the coach station. After we jumped into the back of the car, the first thing I did was light a cigarette, secretly challenging Terry to discipline me. She didn't. Instead, she asked me for one. When she turned around to take her cigarette it was the first time I had seen her face in nine years, and the only thing that matched my memory of her, what I had built her up to be in my mind, were her knowing brown eyes. She wasn't as beautiful as I remembered; perhaps it was because time had been cruel. What bothered me most was the way she kept vacantly laughing like a woman who had gone mad, sounding thick when she spoke too. I felt all my breath full of expectation leaving me heavy and shrunken, my heart contracted in the realisation that she was just a pathetic weak woman who had lost control. The only thing special about her was Tina, Sheila and me.

Shoving my disappointment aside, I asked the one thing I wanted and needed to know — the whole reason for our visit. 'So why didn't you come back and get us from the DU?'

'Ah, you're hung up on the whole DU thing too. That messed with my head for some time.'

'Well?' I said waiting for a real answer.

'I went to court the day I was supposed to see you and they took away permanent custody of you. You were always so upset when I had to leave, clinging to my legs and crying. I couldn't stand telling you the truth and seeing your reaction.'

'Why did you leave us alone in the first place and get yourself into that situation?

'I followed a boyfriend who had left me.'

I mumbled under my breath, 'Well, that's alright then' and blew cigarette smoke in her direction.

Irritated, I then said, 'and who is my real dad, anyway? Every time I turn around I hear a different story.'

'George Bradley'

'Are you sure? Weren't you sleeping with Lawrence Ketler at the time?'

'You and Sheila have the same father. Larry signed the papers and accepted you as his own, but your real father is definitely George. George Hampton Bradley' she said in a somewhat annoyed tone.

Alice looked at me and said, 'Lola...' as if to say that was enough of the third degree.

We drove on in silence.

Alice later wrote:

> I remember when we hung out with your real mom. I think your mom was really drunk but she seemed happy to have her daughters around her. She just acted like you

guys were her old friends or something, though. Not her children.

Tina, who was by now heavily pregnant with her second child, drove us back to her house. We all sat around feeling uncomfortable when Tina went into the kitchen and slipped some cocaine or speed into her drink so Allan wouldn't know. I saw it though. I decided on a whim that I couldn't sit there a moment longer; I felt like the walls were closing in on me and I couldn't breathe. I asked to borrow Tina's phone so I could call some friends that lived in the area. I arranged to meet them at somebody's apartment, and Tina said she would drive Alice and me there. Feeling guilty about leaving Terry so quickly, I invited her along. To my surprise, she came.

She sat with about ten of us while we smoked pot and cigarettes, and some of the guys watched Debbie does Dallas. One of my friends asked me to ask Terry if she would buy us some alcohol, and against my better judgement, I did. After saying she wouldn't, Terry went quiet and moody and then said she was going. She let me believe that she felt used, that we had invited her along just to get some booze, so I felt terrible after she left. I kept telling Alice that I was worried I had hurt her feelings. Alice kept reassuring me the reason she left was not because of what had transpired, that Terry had most likely planned it all along as a way to get away from Tina and Allan long enough to have a drink. I didn't believe her until a couple of days later when Tina rang to say Terry had finally surfaced again after her latest binge at the local bars. I wasn't to see or speak to Terry again for another five years.

Chapter 26

Leaving

Dad tried every trick in the book to convince me to stay. He came upstairs into my room, shut the door and said he would take me off their medical insurance if I left. I continued to pack my belongings.

'You are being very selfish to your sister.' He waited for a reply but got none. 'Lora, can't you see if you leave you are being weak. If you don't learn to face your battles you'll never be able to deal with anything, you'll just keep running. You can't stand up to the real world.'

'I'll deal with my problems – you deal with yours. All the things you just said to me, and have said many times before, don't affect or hurt me anymore. Just go away and leave me alone.'

Dad gave up and left my room, and I sat on my bed for the last time and cried deeply because it really did hurt me very much. He never had faith in me, and that is all I had ever wanted.

The decision to leave my parents' house at sixteen came after a great deal of thought and angst. I had cried so many tears trying to be the daughter they wanted me to be, but nothing I ever did seemed good enough and I was driving myself into the ground trying. When I felt I was making progress, I would then do something wrong and the ravine between us grew wider again. I wanted so much to please them. I sought their love constantly in small and large ways. I prayed to God continually asking him for guidance, to show me how to be a good girl and do everything just as they would like. It seemed they always overlooked every good thing I did, and all their attention went to the smallest of 'wrong' things. Mom had a file in her bedroom documenting everything I did or said wrong. I felt like she was building up a case against me so that one day when they decided to re-home me, they could grab the folder and explain away their decision surrendering all responsibility.

Being my own parent, I wrote a list of goals to follow:

1. *STOP SMOKING – Write in your journal when you feel the need to smoke*

2. *Do my BEST in school*

3. *IMPROVE MY RESPECT TOWARDS OTHERS*

4. *Become more aware of the needs of others*

5. *Spend some more devoted time with my family – take interest in them – **show my love in one way or another to each family member once a day***

6. *BE MYSELF – be consistent and real. Be the same Lora with friends as with family.*

7. *Take responsibility. Do chores without being asked – be home at designated time – do what you say you're going to do*

8. Find a job – eventually – keep in mind things that strike your fancy

It's no wonder I couldn't live up to expectations. I think given that I had just survived cancer and was still spinning from the truth that I might have died was something in itself, not to mention the pain of being abandoned by my biological mother and being taken away from my sisters. The mere fact that I was still there, not giving up, fighting for the right to take my next breath, and struggling to make sense of my muddled and painful childhood should have been enough. I still cared and wanted to behave differently, and my parents should have embraced that, not overlooked or criticized me.

That night I realised I couldn't keep beating myself up and accepted I would never be what my parents wanted. I told them what I intended to do and asked them to please let me leave with dignity instead of sneaking out my window in the night. Begrudgingly they gave me their permission and said they would leave the house during the time I was packing so that my four year old little sister wouldn't witness my leaving. I didn't worry about Kay, though. She had everything she wanted, and by then she was already learning that Lora Lee was a naughty girl. She even started telling me what to do, and how to do it – looking down at me from her short three foot two inches. If I hadn't known Kay was adopted, I would swear on my life that Kay was Mom's biological daughter. They were both short, had dark brown hair, brown eyes and olive skin. What wound me up most was how Kay acted as Mom did towards me – always finding faults in everything I did, and telling on me when I did the slightest thing wrong. In many ways, it often felt like it was Kay and Mom against Dad and me.

As I brought my bags downstairs from my bedroom and loaded up the taxi with my belongings, Mom's sister sat on the couch watching TV. Tears welled in my eyes, and my lips quivered but I refused to cry in front of her. I didn't want anyone to think I was weak or sorry for the decision I had made.

Making my way to a friend's house, in the dark and away from the safety of my parent's home, I sat in the back of the taxi and cried as quietly as I could. Despite all my pain and fear of the unknown, I also had a huge sense of relief wash over me. I no longer had to live up to anybody's expectations but my own. Mom jokes now, 'You're the only girl I know that would ring a taxi to run away from home!' I never realised my own expectations would be the most demanding of all.

For a couple of months I stayed with various friends who eventually asked me to leave. One friend I stayed with had a large room in a house big enough to be a Hollywood actor's home. It was ideal. I couldn't believe my luck until she took the Hollywood actor thing too far and started using cocaine. Living near San Francisco, LSD was an almost necessary experience – like it was written in my adolescent growing up manual that because I lived near the infamous Haight Street, I must try LSD at least once. Cocaine, speed, crack and heroine, however, are all drugs a step too far for me, so I never got involved. I just watched my friend slowly nearly kill herself.

Her behaviour became more and more erratic. One evening whilst I sat on her couch in her bedroom flipping through Vogue, she sat at her desk cutting cocaine. I think she was adding something to it to make it heavier so she could sell it for more money. Something went wrong and she screamed that it was all fucking wasted. I sat quietly as she tore up her room in frustration. Then she turned on me, 'Get out! Get the fuck out and never come back!' She grabbed and threw my things at me. So just like that I was once again homeless. A couple of months later I heard she was in rehab, which was a relief to learn as I'm certain she would have killed herself carrying on the way she was.

At one point I stayed with my boyfriend in his rented room. After a couple of weeks, he also gave me my walking papers saying he was embarrassed and tired of the responsibility of taking care of me. I went clubbing and wrote the following note to myself that evening, Thanksgiving night:

> I want to have a home. I'm scared. I'd be fine if there weren't so many things holding me back. I want to crawl away and die. There are so many tears held within me... Is this the beginning of something wonderful, or the end? I still want to run away, but I already am. I'm at Das Klub (in San Francisco) – wanna dance this shit out of me. Bye.

In the end, I exhausted all my options and was contemplating living rough when, as if by another act of God, my friend Wendy and her mother were kind enough to allow me to share a room with Wendy, eat their food, and treat their house as if it was mine. They didn't even ask me to pay rent. Finally, with a bit of stability around me, I was able to find a job and worked full time at an Acrylic Design and Fabrication shop.

Wendy and I got on well for the most part. She was an artistic soul who found expression through her unique vintage dress style, the music she listened to, and her room where she displayed her colourful artwork from ceiling to floor.

When I went home for Christmas that year, as soon as I walked through my parent's door, Mom asked me to follow her into her bedroom; she had something she needed to tell me. Once she shut the door, she nervously began, 'You know I have wanted a baby of my own for nearly twenty years...'

I nodded yes.

'I'm pregnant!'

I was so happy for her I cried. For years I had prayed that God would give the one thing she wanted so much. I gave her a bear hug and told her how pleased I was for her and Dad. We went back out and joined the rest of the family and shared the good news.

Back at Wendy's and work I was learning what it was like to be an adult with responsibilities. I bought myself a moped to get to and from work, and I was proud of myself for how well I was doing. Despite all my advances, I felt a constant fear that the police would pick me up and take me back to Hillcrest Juvenile Hall because technically I was still a minor and runaway.

Alice continued to live between Oregon and the San Francisco Bay Area, and Wendy and I continued to be very close friends. In fact, in the end, it was as if we were sisters, always bickering and competing but very protective and supportive at the same time. I was eighteen months older than her, and I believe it frustrated her that I got to go clubbing while she had to stay home. Alice visited on the odd occasion, but it wasn't the same. She now had closer friends, and regrettably so did I.

Then it happened. One morning on the way to work a policeman pulled me over on my moped. He seemed to know who I was and what he thought he was dealing with and looking for. He went through my handbag inspecting every tube of lipstick and makeup compact. He even felt the lining of my bag and appeared most disappointed when he didn't find the drugs he was looking for; the drugs he would never find because I no longer used drugs of any sort.

When the policeman ran my name in his computer I came up as

a runaway, and was asked to sit in the back of his car. I had no idea where he was taking me and I watched life flick by like a book of animations as we drove along. I wondered if I would ever be free like everybody else just to live and be myself. I was so frightened they'd put me back into the social care system and once again I'd be somebody's parcel to do with as they liked. I held my stomach as waves of queasiness came over me and I imagined all my hard efforts going unnoticed and being wasted.

Back at Hillcrest Juvenile Hall, I sat in my cell feeling panic and stress. *Oh God, will I ever be free? Why do they keep insisting on controlling me? All I want is my freedom to live the way I want to.* Suddenly David, a member of staff I knew from previous visits, came into my room. He was really happy to see me, asking me how I was and what I had been up to. I updated him and when I got to the part where the police had stopped me and taken me into custody, I said, 'I should have run, or I should have lied about who I was. I wouldn't be here now if I had.' David chuckled warmly and said that was how criminals think, and I definitely wasn't a criminal. Before leaving he reassured me I had done the right thing and felt only good would come out of it. I always liked David because he seemed to have so much faith in me.

He was right, too. The following morning, I sat in court listening to someone represent my case, and to my surprise it was decided that because I had proven for over six months to be responsible, drug free and not causing any trouble, I should be emancipated and considered an adult capable of caring for myself.

I walked away that day feeling like I had reached a milestone in my life. At the age of 16 I was now officially a respectable adult. I held my head up high and breathed in the scents around me a little more deeply. I always knew freedom would be so sweet and intoxicating.

Within a couple of months, I regrettably left Wendy's and moved into my own apartment without even saying how thankful and indebted I was to her and her mother. I was very lucky they had come to my rescue when they did. If it weren't for that miracle, I would have been living on the street, and emancipation from the court and my parents may not have been possible.

Chapter 27

An irresponsible adult

Not long after proving myself a responsible adult, I was fired for being late to work. It doesn't sound like such a major thing, but it happened on a day I was in charge, and I didn't arrive to work with the front door key until 12:00 PM while the other employees had been waiting since 9:00 AM.

Instead of going out and looking for another job, I rang Sheila who I hadn't seen in eight years and asked her to fly out and visit me – my treat. Nothing like living for the day and being irresponsible.

Sheila visited; Tina was invited and visited too, and we partied in my apartment with my many friends. Because I was such a 'Wild Child' and lived for the moment, I didn't slow down enough to appreciate it was the first time us three girls had been together since the DU in Santa Rosa. I was in full swing social mode, serving drinks, smoking and behaving as if I had just won an Oscar. We were having a jolly time when Look Alike Nick, (my still gay first boyfriend I was now friendly with), and Sheila got into a bitchy catfight. Sheila was saying how much she cared and wanted to be there for me during my cancer treatment. Look Alike Nick (who still looked the same) said, 'Then why weren't you?'

Sheila retorted, 'Honey, don't you be messing with me.'

'Look Honey, all I'm saying is you had a choice.'

I shouted for both of them to shut up stating, 'Neither of you were there for me and you both could have been. You are both as bad as the other.' Look alike Nick sneered some at Sheila, and Sheila changed the subject.

Later that night, after a copious amount of booze was consumed, Tina and Sheila started talking about the past. What started as talking soon became red faces, snotty noses, floods of tears, and neither one listening as the other ranted. They were fighting over who hurt the most because of our past. I stayed out of it not out of politeness but because for me it was no contest. I implored for both of them to please make up and stop their fighting. Eventually they jumped up off the floor and told me they were driving to Tina's house two hours away in Santa Rosa. Not the most sensible thing to do considering how much alcohol had been drunk. Looking a little worse for wear, they didn't return until the next day. Whatever happened that night remains their secret.

Eventually I got another job. Indeed, I would have several jobs over the next couple of years, but the one that stands out most is Macys Department Store at Hillsdale Mall. I worked in the Junior Department as a full time sales assistant where I met Jill who was what we called a 'floater.' No, she wasn't a big brown floating turd! She was a 'floater' because she floated from department to department helping when other staff members were ill. She was to become a life long friend.

I lived in a one-bedroom apartment in Burlingame and my little sister Kay, now seven, would come and stay the night with me from time to time. My brother William had arrived and although

I didn't find it difficult to accept him, I could see it was hard on Kay. Every time I called or visited it was, 'Will this' and 'Will that,' and Kay was used to being the centre of attention. Therefore, I tried to create a special place for her to get undivided attention.

I loved Kay, but I found our visits difficult because: Number 1 – She judged me. She wouldn't even eat the food I cooked for her because she had it in her mind that everything associated with me was tainted – including the pancakes I'd cook her for breakfast. Number 2 – She was emotionally unstable and challenging, and I found this very difficult to deal with. One moment she would be laughing hysterically, and the next she was sitting in a despondent manner, looking at a spot on the ground deep in thought. She would never talk about what she was experiencing and her mood changed frequently, so it was quite exhausting trying to keep up with her tribulations. None the less, I continued to have her around because I wanted to have some resemblance of a relationship with her even though I had moved out of my parents' house. I ended up being like a second mother to her.

I had many boyfriends. When one relationship ended, usually because I had that lost that loving feeling, I went straight on to the next guy without a moment's hesitation. When I look back and read my old journals, what strikes me most is my need to be loved. Without even realising it, I was repeating Terry's behaviour. Terry once told me that her father never said he loved her before he died, so it's no wonder she went from man to man looking for the love she felt she was missing. Right or wrong, I didn't feel loved, so I looked to boys for the unconditional love I felt I needed from them.

I never realised the love I needed most was the love from me to me, the love I should have learned as a child. If Terry had loved, protected, cherished and cared for me – I would have grown up with the belief that I was a person worth loving. As it was, I apologised to everybody for needing his or her love and affection, and still find myself doing it to this day.

One boyfriend, Mr Artist, who I was especially fond of, disappeared off to the California College of Arts and Crafts and suddenly for the one of the first times in my life I was on my own. Although I found it an extremely painful time, it was also very healing. It gave me time to reflect and decide what was important to me. Not wishing to be left behind, I subsequently enrolled in college full time, moved into my parent's garage to save money and found myself a full time job to support myself and pay off my credit card bills. I enjoyed getting straight A's and the social aspect of campus life. Before long I was dating the president of student services, Mr Social, smiley nice guy who was cheerfulness personified, and was a regular at the school's 'cool' café in between classes. Once again, I felt like my life was settling down and I could just about smile again. Wendy and I were even considering going to England and studying through a division of London University.

Chapter 28

A visit 'back East'

During a half term break from college, I made a trip to the east coast to visit Sheila whom I hadn't seen for three years. Her youngest daughter was ten months old, and her two eldest daughters were four and five. She lived with her first husband who it became clear had a drug problem, and had a boyfriend on the side to make up for her husband's inadequacies. Her two-bedroom house was modest and sweet. Her strong artistic streak inherited from Terry meant she was able to make and create almost anything. As a result, her home had warmth and a unique Raggedy Ann and Andy country style to it. It was fun to be in her environment. I slept on one of her daughter's beds, and Sheila snuck in late one night before going to bed so we could play racing cars one more time just for memories sake.

Whilst visiting Sheila, Tina heard I was there and got on a Grey Hound bus and made her way across the United States to be with us. We all met up at Terry's house for an impromptu family reunion. It was the first time we were all together with Terry since the DU. Terry clung to me, licking my face like a cat and in disgust I told her to knock it off as I wiped her saliva from my cheek. She said something about me being her baby kitten, and I shuddered in disgust. She moved away from me and I sat on her couch taking in the usual décor: beer signs, tacky cat pictures, a large velour picture of Elvis, and framed puzzles hanging on her wall.

When Tina arrived with no bags to speak of, wearing only a vest and a red baseball cap, she was already drunk and had numerous bruises on her upper body. We all sat and talked whilst we drank beer. Inevitably somebody brought up the past, and suddenly Terry turned on me, 'You don't think I raised you? Who do you think changed your diapers?'

'You certainly didn't,' I defiantly replied.

I was lucky she let that one slide. If it had been Sheila or Tina, a huge verbal and maybe even physical fight would have ensued.

Further into the evening, Terry went into the loo and suddenly, as if in pain, we heard her shouting for us – asking us to come quickly. She was sat on the toilet in the dark with her pants down around her ankles. She said, 'I just wanted you guys to know how sorry I am about what happened.' She was weeping, 'I love you guys so much…'

Sheila burst out in a fit of laughter and quipped, 'Is that it? We've been waiting all our lives for that speech? You sat drunk on a toilet saying you love us? Damn!'

We all burst into laughter.

Conscious of keeping control of what could easily be an explosive situation, Sheila and I left shortly thereafter. Tina stayed with Terry and continued drinking.

The next morning, Sheila telephoned Terry and found out that after we left she and Tina had an enormous argument, ending with Tina smashing Terry's front door glass pane with her fist, and leaving in the middle of the night. Nobody knew where Tina was.

Hearing the news, the first thing Sheila and I did was drive to Terry's, and whilst I was clearing up all the glass at the front door, her neighbour appeared. The woman remarked how noisy it had been the previous night, and asked what happened to the front door. For some reason I protected Terry by lying, 'Oh, when we left last night I slammed the door too hard – I was drunk. Didn't know my own strength.' As soon as I said it, I questioned my motives. Did I still see Terry as an extension of myself even now?

Sheila knew exactly where to look for Tina – the local bars. We drove to one; Sheila left me in the car and came back out in a matter of minutes. 'Yeah, she's been here, but left with *some man*.' Sheila also knew where this man lived and we made our way there. Once again I waited in the car.

Sheila was gone for about half an hour before reappearing with a very worse for wear Tina. She had found her passed out on a bare mattress on the floor of an empty room. Once we were all safely in the car, Sheila and Tina immediately started arguing. Sheila couldn't believe Tina was sleeping on a pissed on old mattress with a man she didn't even know. Tina defended herself by saying, 'What do you care? You haven't even tried to find me these past few years. All you care about is yourself.'

Trying to pick the right moment, I eventually interjected asking Sheila if Tina could come back to hers, and Sheila reluctantly agreed. When we arrived at Sheila's, I insisted Tina take a bath and drew the water for her. I then proceeded to undress and help her into the bath. Frightened she might go under if I left her alone, I sat by her side until she finished. I gave her some of my clothes to wear, and we all settled down to watch TV and rest.

A couple of days later I was due to fly home, and when it came time to leave for the airport, Tina said, 'Oh, I guess you want your clothes back.' I told her to forget about it. She laughed and said, 'I knew you'd say that!'

Chapter 29

A fresh beginning

Because I was dating Mr Social, smiley nice guy who was cheerfulness personified and didn't want to leave him on his own for more than a second because he couldn't keep his trousers zipped up, Wendy went to England without me. Slowly I got tired of waking up to happy notes reminding me to wake up happy and smile, or maybe I just got tired of smiling through gritted teeth, but the end result was that I went to England the following semester leaving him behind after nearly two years of dating.

I will never understand my driving ambition to go to England. From the time I was a young girl, England was something I spoke of as much as Elvis or boys. When I boarded the plane at San Francisco International Airport, there was a real mix of excitement and fear of the unknown. The whole plane was full of students my age about to embark on making dreams come true, believing that going to England would somehow change their life, and I certainly count myself as one of them. The girl next to me was dowdy, wore no makeup, was about 100 pounds overweight, and her shoulder length poodle curly hair zinged off in every direction. She was quiet and shy, so we didn't speak much for the duration of the flight.

Half way through the journey I fell asleep with my Walkman on, and when I awoke, I opened the window and looked out at the rising radiant sun peering just above the edge of the clouds. Rod Stewart's song, *Sailing* had just started, and as he sang the words, *I am flying. I am flying. Like a bird, cross the sky. I am flying, across the high clouds, to be near you, to be free.* I nearly wept. I felt like for once in my life I knew where I was going, and a deep part of me did feel like I was coming home – that I had been here before.

Funded by a student grant and armed with Mom's credit card, I lived in a building full of other Americans at Cornwall Gardens, Kensington and studied English through a division of London University. In particular, I enjoyed going to show after show, learning how to write reviews. It was fun; I had a load of American friends to keep me company, and the whole experience felt more like a party than school.

One evening after the pubs had closed, a couple of girlfriends and I made our way to a club called Hombres in London. We sat at the bar nursing our gin and tonics when I noticed a tall, slender man with short, dark hair meeting my eye. My girlfriend stood between him and me with her back to me trying to hit on him, asking him loads of questions, and each time he answered with, 'So, whose your friend?' looking in my direction and smiling.

Eventually my friend became so frustrated she said, 'Oh for God's sake – that's Lora!' and walked away flipping her irritation out of her hair.

He made his way over to me and speaking over the loud music said, 'Hello Lora. I'm James.'

We chatted into the night and I learned he was a police constable who had worked with the Metropolitan police for three years. I was impressed that a guy as young as I could be so responsible and stable. Most of the young guys I had dated in the States were still living at home with no idea of what they wanted to do for a career. James' independence, stability, and charm caught my imagination, and my 'Wild Child' once again took over the controls.

After a month or so of living and breathing one another, I heard the words, 'Do you, Miss Wild Child, take Mr Responsible and Stable to be your lawfully wedded husband?' Then, as if in another dimension, I heard 'Wild Child' say, 'I do.' And just like that, we were married.

In all honesty, I did have my reservations the evening before I married James. I laid awake thinking of the ceremony to follow the next morning at the Registry Office in Chelsea. I rationalised away all common sense. I knew I really liked him, I thought he was handsome, but I didn't feel the way I thought I would when I got married. There were no butterflies, common interests, or a long history to speak of, and in retrospect, I question if I even loved him. I was only 21; I didn't even know what love was. I had tried to find it all my young but full life and each time I was spectacularly disappointed.

In the end, I told myself that there was no such thing as the love I had in mind, that James was a good catch. He had a good job, was handsome and secure. A girl like me would be a fool to pass him up. I mean all the other girls in my building fancied him. I decided just to take the jump and marry him. I knew it meant commitment, and I was ready to give it a go. I thought of the movie *Moonstruck* starring Cher where she told a relative that she was getting married and they asked, 'Do you love him?' to which she replied, 'No.' They said, 'Good. It never works when you love them.'

James and I made a real go of it, though. We started by making a disastrous start. After my term had finished in college, I flew home with the other students. I sat next to the same girl I had on the way to England, and I smiled inwardly when I saw the difference in her even after just four months. She had lost about fifty pounds, wore bright red lipstick, a tight purple leotard shirt and her hair was conditioned and styled into a very trendy cut. She was full of life and I couldn't get two words in edgewise. That was OK, though. I had many things on my mind like *where will I live when I get back to the States?* And, *what on earth do I tell my parents who don't even know what I've done?*

The first question was answered when Mom asked if I would be moving back into the garage. 'Yes! Of course I am' (phew – thank God that was easy.) It gave me an opportunity to work and save money for James and me to rent a place. We were only 21- James didn't even have enough money to buy me an engagement ring let alone a house. Having floated around my mind for three months, the second question was answered when James came for a visit and Mom told me he had to sleep in a different room because we weren't married. I told her sheepishly, 'err....ummmm... actually Mom, we are...' looking away, avoiding her eyes and reaction as I said it.

Mom said, 'Well you know what Kay is like. She'll want to see the certificate; otherwise, she won't believe you.' In other words, Mom thought I was lying to get my way and wanted to see the marriage certificate herself. I showed her, and she looked at it in disbelief. I think she was angry but didn't say so. This was one of those moments where my parents showed great restraint by not saying anything except to ask if I really wanted a white wedding since we were already married. Of course I did! Absolutely. I needed my moment in the spotlight. I wanted my fairytale beginning.

After a year or so of writing each other and the odd visit, James took time off from his work in the UK to join me in California. In anticipation of his arrival, I had moved into a one-bedroom apartment and had quit smoking because I knew it bothered him. It was I who paid the deposit and first couple of month's rent in addition to funding all the furnishings. Angry that he had enough money for endless nights at the pub back in England and an expensive Marin mountain bicycle that he bought in the States and took back with him, I decided it was high time he contributed to our household. I took his credit card number and charged him $500 through my parent's business and they gave me cash in return. When James found out, we had a spectacular argument about money; one of many that were to follow.

Whilst waiting for James to join me, I made several road trips to see Sheila and her boyfriend-cum-husband Dale in Vista, near San Diego where he was stationed. Dale was a Master Gunnery Sergeant in the Marines so they lived with Sheila's three daughters in an apartment complex full of other Marines and their families. Sheila started an adult education program to get her high school diploma. Although her life long aspiration was to join the Marines, this was never a realistic proposition because she had so many little ones dependent on her. Unfortunately it wasn't long before Sheila and her family moved back to North Carolina and our visits stopped.

James worked for my parents cleaning carpets, while I, having long since left college with only an AA degree, worked as a secretary for a water-engineering firm. Both jobs paid rather well, and we were living comfortably. On the surface everything appeared hunky dory. Behind closed doors, however, the cracks were beginning to show and our arguments intensified.

The fairytale wedding took place a year and 10 days after our first civil ceremony in England. It was December 20 when James and I stood before the Reverend of my parent's church and my hands shook under the weight of my lily bouquet. Sheila was my maid of honour, and friends Jill and Wendy and little sister Kay were my bride's maids. I rang Alice several times whilst living as a student in England, and she never returned my calls, so although I invited her to my wedding, I didn't feel it was appropriate to ask her to be a bride's maid. I have no idea where Tina was during this time. She always disappeared when things were really out of control in her life, and Terry wasn't there for the simple reason she wasn't invited – not that she would have attended anyway. Nobody except James' mother attended from his side of the family, not that they couldn't afford to, so we asked Jill's husband, my father, and a friend of my parents to act as James' best men, and my brother William to be the ring bearer. It was a hugely beautiful and expensive wedding. Looking back at the photos, it was definitely the white wedding every little girl dreams of.

The reception was joyous too. It was a perfect dreamy day. James and I arrived at our hotel room with smiles from ear to ear and started talking about our wedding and reception full of excitement. I said, 'Oh my God, I never knew Ed could dance like that! He and Sheila were amazing.'

'Yeah, I think I married the wrong sister.'

'What?'

'When we were leaving a video message she kept running her hand up and down my leg.'

'She was drunk.'

'Yeah, but still – I imagine she was up for it.'

This conversation was definitely not scripted into my fairytale wedding, and not the best thing to say to the bride on her wedding night, especially not a bride who had drunk too much wine. I went into the bathroom, slammed the door and locked it. Oh dear, it looked like another disastrous start.

The next disaster came the following morning when James and I, his mother, Sheila, her three girls and two teenage girls from my parent's church all went on our honeymoon to Lake Tahoe together. Upon our arrival at the cabin, Sheila and James' mother had to share a room, and immediately began fighting. June called Sheila a slut saying that it meant something different in the UK and Sheila replied, 'At least I'm not old!'

Approximately a year after our white wedding, James and I decided to move back to the UK so he could start working in the police force again. He went ahead of me to try to find us a flat, and I stayed back for a couple of months to save more money and organise the shipping of all our possessions, which luckily were very few because once again it was me who had to pay.

What I didn't ship I gave to Tina and her boyfriend who she'd met through AA meetings. He and Tina drove off in his black pick up truck full of all my possessions toppling over like Dr Seuss's character Cat in a Hat precariously balancing a stack of fine china. Swallowing hard and hoping I had made the right decision, I questioned if I was only running like Terry always did, outdoing her this time by not only leaving the state but an entire country. Was Dad right: would I ever be able to face reality and deal with my problems? Was I being weak?

I confused all these thoughts with what could have been a genuine leap of faith to be with my husband. Was I just insecure and fearful of being perceived as following in Terry's footsteps, or was there some validity to my concerns? My mind worked overtime on finding answers to these questions as I watched everything I had acquired and made my life to be, being driven away from me. I decided perhaps it was a little of both, and filed the thoughts away somewhere deep inside, tightening my lips once again and making every conscious effort to move on. The consequences would be what they would be.

Before joining James in England, I aged 23, attended an antenatal appointment because I had missed two periods and a home pregnancy test said I was pregnant. Half of me was worried what James would say and the other half of me hoped it was true. Whilst the doctor scanned me to verify my pregnancy, I asked if it was possible to tell what gender it was. The nurse started, 'At this point, only a few weeks along it would be very…' her words hung in the air before she said, 'Do you really want to know? I have a very clear image here.' I crossed my fingers and toes, made my wish and said, 'Yes!' She moved the monitor around so I could see, and as clear as day, there was my first child with its legs spread eagled. Smile for the camera, son. My sweet little boy – just what I wanted. I vowed as I watched life wriggle inside me, that I would protect and love him to a fault — my first-born, a piece of my heart.

A couple of weeks before I embarked on a new voyage to distant lands, Mom threw me a baby shower with her best friend who was also expecting. It would be the last time I would see my close friends for some time so it also served as a goodbye and good luck party.

When I agreed to move to England, I had visions of how it had been previously. I thought I would have many friends around for emotional support and companionship, that I would live in a lovely area in a beautiful block of flats and would travel into central London frequently to enjoy a show and a meal, and would have an endless supply of cash to buy what I needed when I needed it. But the day I arrived in England with every last possession packed into two suitcases, James took me back to the very modest flat he rented for us in Shortlands near Bromley,

Kent. When I saw my new home for the first time, I had my first *Oh Dear* moment. The flat was tiny and simple. It was furnished with MDF furniture, had cheap carpets, two small rooms and bathrooms, and a very tiny kitchen that could just about withstand two people in it at the same time. There was no dining room, so I had to put a table in our lounge, making what was a small room feel even smaller. Although the flat was clean and modern, I immediately felt disappointed — like how I have felt previously when I arrived at a hotel room and realised I was going to have to spend an entire holiday there. Take that feeling and combine it with the next thought, *it will never end – I'll always be here,* and you may come close to experiencing the dread beginning to brew deep inside.

Disappointed, I asked, 'James, do you have any bubble bath so I can have a soak?'

He didn't, but said he was going to the store and would pick me up some along with some conditioner for my hair. Knowing him fairly well by now, I said, 'Please promise me you won't buy the cheapest products in the store.'

'Now would I do that?' he asked cheekily.

While he was gone I went through the flat looking at the photos of him and me that he had framed, stared out the window at the communal garden below and watched rain streak down the window. The combination of rain and my reflection staring back at me made it look like I was crying. I thought *how appropriate* as I tried to reassure myself things would get better.

On James' return I started to draw a bath and pour in some of the blue fluid that was supposed to be bubble bath. 'Oh James! This smells like cheap men's cologne. It's disgusting. You've done it again – you bought the cheapest you could find.'

'What's wrong with it?' James asked seriously.

'What, besides it stinking like Old Spice? It's as thin as water.'

In the bath I sniffed at the shampoo and realised it wasn't any better. It stunk of artificial strawberries, and the conditioner left my hair feeling like straw. At least in the States I had my own income and could afford the finer things that made my life more enjoyable. I could see I was going to learn a completely new way of life with James.

As I was five months pregnant, and unable to understand most English, Irish, and Scottish accents, I couldn't work before my son was born. As a result, I had nowhere to go each day, no friends, no family nearby, no money, no car and a husband who worked so much overtime I never saw him. I didn't even benefit from the extra money he earned; he kept his own bank account that I had no access to. In fact, everything was in his name and he had all control over every aspect of my life. If I wanted to buy a pair of knickers, I had to ask his permission. If I wanted a haircut, I had to either go to one he would pay for (£6 or less), or I had to delve into the last little bit of American money I still had left. When I asked for money to buy some stationary to write my family and friends, he said he would get it for me. He brought me home Metropolitan Police letterhead. I felt confined, controlled, bored, friendless, pregnant, penniless and miserable from day one.

I wrote my family and friends constantly in the beginning, but never had any replies so eventually gave up. Although I did see Wendy and Jill during visits home, unfortunately I lost touch with Alice.

I was rushed to the hospital early in the morning on a spring day, and after 21 hours of sheer agony, I gave birth to a pale grey and lifeless baby. It never once occurred to me that something could go wrong until I watched the midwife pump his legs vigorously. Another midwife vigilantly rubbed him all over with a soft white towel. I held my breath as they tried desperately to get a response from my newborn. I kept asking, 'Is he all right? Is he OK? What's happening?' and they pretended not to hear as they mechanically went through an algorithm of what to do when a baby is unresponsive at birth. As I escalated into complete hysteria, and just before I nearly lost it altogether, my son took his first huge gulp of air and let out an enormous loud cry. Colour filled his body and life was restored to my face. I never thought a baby's cry could be so wonderful.

The following day I left the hospital for home with Peter James (PJ) bundled like a little Eskimo in my arms. As I looked down at the sun shining on his perfectly squashed face, I thought, *you're really going to let me walk away with this precious life? You trust me enough?*

Mom had already been staying with us for ten days before being present during the delivery of PJ; therefore, she didn't have much time to spend with us following his birth before she had to go home to Dad, Kay and William. Knowing she was due to leave soon, I stood in my little kitchen on the fifth floor of our building looking out at the large conker tree across the street. Full of hormones, I burst into tears at the thought that I would be left alone in a strange country without her help and support.

James had already gone back to work the day after PJ was born, and after Mom left I had a uterine infection causing me chills, sweats and hallucinations. I feared I wouldn't be able to cope and that my depression would get the worst of me, but luckily the fever soon passed and I quickly learned how to be a mother. In fact, motherhood came quite naturally and I found that I was good at it. Every time I looked at PJ in the first few months I asked myself how any woman could ever leave her child. I had only been his mother a very short time, and already would have sacrificed my life for his. How could a woman leave not one, but three of her children after years of raising them?

Chapter 30

Accepting a hard truth

After living in the flat in Shortlands for two years, I managed to convince James to move us to Biggin Hill into one of the old RAF Officer's accommodations that had just become available to rent. It wasn't ideal, but at least it had a garden for my son, a place for me to plant flowers, and after I worked hard painting and decorating the inside, it felt like a home.

I worked full time at an Alcohol Advisory Service as a PA to the Director and in the evenings trained as an Alcohol Counsellor to complement our modest income. All the women I worked with were much older than I was, so I forged no close friendships. I did have one good friend that I made through James' friend (also a police constable), but I was always conscious of not smothering or suffocating her with my neediness. James still worked night and day; I hardly ever saw him, and when I did, he usually told me to shut up because he was watching TV, or we argued about anything and everything.

Lonely and bored, I rang his work one evening, and the person on duty told me he had already signed out hours before. When I questioned if he was sure, he laughed and told me he was positive. When I asked James about it, he said he had been at work, that it was all a misunderstanding. I chose to believe him because frankly by that point I didn't care much either way.

Sheila came to England for the first time just before PJ's third birthday and we planned to go for five days on a last minute deal to Majorca. James suddenly announced he was going fishing with some mates and I had to take PJ with me. It made our trip a lot less fun, that's for sure.

On our arrival back, it was a lovely warm spring day so Sheila and I sat in my garden while PJ napped. James rolled up in a car full of men, got out with his Armani Suit hanging from a hanger in one hand. Sheila looked at me with raised eyebrows and a, *what the hell?* expression. I asked James why he had his suit with him to go fishing, and he defiantly replied, 'I took a fish to my mother in it.' And, guess what? I believed him. To this day, Sheila says she was tempted to hit me over the head with a frying pan to make me see clearly again. I still don't know exactly why he was lying, but I can certainly guess.

The first visit back to the States I made with James and PJ. We stayed with my parents and slept in my old bedroom, and amongst other outings and days out, I decided I wanted to visit Tina and her boyfriend. Tina, her boyfriend, two children and I spent the day together at the San Francisco zoo. James refused to go because he didn't approve of associating himself with 'criminals.' Instead, he took a daylong tour of San Francisco by himself. When he arrived back to my parent's house that evening, he was sun burned and I felt secretly happy believing it was karma repaying him for being such a pompous prat towards my sister.

The second time I visited the States I went on my own with PJ for a month. This time Tina came without her boyfriend to visit me at my parent's house. We went to the San Jose flea market together, where Tina began talking about another man named

Luis. I knew my sister well enough to know she had fallen for Luis, and I was worried because she told me he drank and did drugs, and I knew her mixing with him would lead to only one outcome. I expressed my concerns to her, and she said, 'I know,' but I seriously doubted she did.

On my return to the UK from my visit abroad, I felt full of despair to be back in the same situation with James. It never got any better and there was no promise that it ever would. Days became months of waiting for a glimmer of hope that never appeared. I repeatedly asked James when we would have our own home, and he always replied, 'If you want your own home, get it yourself.'

I would go shopping for food, and he would look over the receipt and delete any items he wouldn't have purchased before reimbursing me the difference. Even though we were by no means skint and there wasn't a drought, he told me to use my dirty dish water to water my plants. I'd turn on the boiler to heat water for a bath and when I'd get in would scream in shock when I registered how cold it was. James had shut off the boiler before the water even had time to heat up.

The hardest aspect of my relationship with James was the relationship he had with his mother. He always put her first, and that caused major stress in our marriage. That, coupled with the fact that she and I never saw eye to eye on how to raise my son, meant James took my baby away from me for long weekends to be with his mother. Left at home away from my son, I would stew over the injustice.

Things continued to deteriorate and I lost hope. One day, I lay curled up in the sunshine at the foot of our bed crying because I realised I had to face a very hard truth. Feeling as if life was passing me by, I looked longingly out of our bedroom window. I was so lonely, overlooked, and caged with no prospects for the future, and I knew there was still a chance at life out there somewhere... somehow. I had to believe I might still find love and happiness. I accepted that after six years, my marriage to James was over.

Leaving James was one of the hardest things I've ever had to do. I loved him in the end, even though I also hated him equally – if not more. I had devoted everything to making our marriage work and leaving him was like grieving over the death of a child or best friend. Most importantly, it was the death of a family for my son. Although I knew it was necessary to leave James to move forward and live again, I felt my heart bleed seeing him cry and asking me to sleep next to him just one more night. I couldn't. I truly wanted to, but knew it would only perpetuate the agony we felt. Instead I walked away crying for all our losses.

Somewhere in between my visits to the States and leaving James, I received a few telephone calls from Tina. At first, she told me how happy she was with Luis, and that she was expecting another baby. The next call she said Luis was 'using' and she wanted to get away from him; could she come stay with me for a bit? James obviously said no. The third call she asked me if I thought she should abort her baby, if that was the solution to her predicament. I said it wasn't a decision for me to make, but if it were I would keep my baby. I had no more phone calls after that.

PJ and I moved into a very modest flat in Surrey. I worked as a Marketing Assistant for a large American air conditioning company, and balanced work with single parenthood rather well. I also met a couple of friends that I would lunch with at work, but they were never the kind of friendships I had with the likes of Alice, Wendy or Jill – all of whom knew how I was feeling before I even spoke. These new friends were fun and the friendships superficial, but for a while that was all I needed and wanted.

The first Christmas with just PJ and me, we travelled to North Carolina to spend it with Sheila and her family. Whilst visiting, Sheila arranged another family get together with her husband and daughters, Terry, Tina, Luis, and her third youngest child Luis. They all lived in North Carolina. Tina had lost touch with her two eldest children who still lived with their father in California, so unfortunately they were not present.

We all met up at a local restaurant. The evening started well, in fact it was fun. For a brief period, we all pretended that the past didn't exist and we were one large and happy family. Terry bought PJ an infant's feeding spoon (he was three years old) and gave me one of her sweaters, which smelled distinctly of vanilla. It saddened me that she had nothing else to give but the clothes off her back.

We laughed and joked, and even Terry and Tina were getting along. Terry made a real effort not drink too much and the evening was ending on a pleasant note. With the bill already settled, we hugged and said our good byes when Terry suddenly became very emotional and asked the waiter for another beer. She managed to keep us all there for another twenty minutes while she finished her drink, but in the end we had to go. I could see how pained both Terry and Tina were as we left. I felt relieved that we managed to get through a meal without the two of them fighting and without the past being brought up.

I decided on a whim whilst visiting Sheila that I wanted to drive to Memphis Tennessee to see Elvis' house, Graceland. I invited Terry, who happily agreed to come along, and then I invited Tina and Luis who also wanted to go. When Terry found out Tina was going, she decided she didn't want to come after all, saying 'I can't handle that shit right now.' I rented a car, and off we went with our two children, bags, and a cooler full of beer.

Every stop we made Tina and Luis bought a couple of beers each, and when we had to cross through a point where it was illegal to sell or consume alcohol, Tina and Luis broke into my supply of beer in the car. When we arrived to Memphis during the night on the second day of our trip, we drank more beer than imaginable. The next morning, before we went to Graceland, we stopped at a café across the road where Tina and Luis had beer for breakfast. By the time we made it to Graceland, Tina was half drunk and tried climbing over the ropes in hopes of stealing upstairs to see Elvis' bedroom. When she was stopped by security, I turned a hundred different shades of red in embarrassment as other tourists named and shamed her.

Despite all the drinking, I enjoyed our trip to Graceland. It was something I had always wanted to do. Even at the age of 27, I felt like a little girl again as I stood staring through thick glass at Elvis' famous white fringed all-in-one suit with the cape full of gems. I don't care what people say, when you see how slim his clothes were, he wasn't as fat as he appeared on TV. As I stood there trying to imagine Elvis filling his own shoes, I realised it would be the closest I would ever come to meeting my idol man. I was close enough to touch and smell the clothes and him, but as usual in my life an invisible barrier was stopping me.

Shortly after my return from North Carolina, I started dating the Commercial Director of the company I worked at. My 'Wild Child' was still at the controls, and the Commercial Director and I moved in together after a matter of months. We rented a town house in Kent for a while before deciding on a whim one day that we would go and look at a house in East Sussex. We went, we saw, and we bought the same day… nothing like living for the moment! It was fun, but deep down I didn't feel comfortable.

Buying my first home was something huge that should have been worked towards. It made me appreciate the gesture a little less, because it seemed so hasty and unimportant to him.

The Commercial Director was tall, blond with blue eyes, and a big build. He was attractive, but it was his confidence and take-charge demeanour that made me look twice. He was used to being in control down to the smallest detail. For instance, he would often pick out my suits for me to wear to work the following day. During business and social engagements, I was expected to stand behind him while he spoke, to only speak when spoken to, and eat what he put on my plate. When he listened to others speak, he continually clenched his jaw impatiently waiting for them to finish, and would laugh too loud before making his excuses and moving onto his next audience. I would smile sweetly and follow like I had no choice. In the beginning this was great because it took the burden off; I didn't have to take any responsibility – even for my own actions. I could remain in my cell and still have a life without having to work for it.

When the Commercial Director and I moved from Kent to East Sussex, all of my friendships ended because it was simply too far for any of them to make an effort to keep in touch, and once again, I got tired of trying. We lived in our new house for a year when PJ started school and I started working as Marketing Assistant at a local company. For a year-and-a-half I worked in that capacity reporting directly to the MD, Peter.

Peter was 39 when I met him at interview. He was tall, slender, had thick dark brown hair and blue eyes. He was strikingly good looking, and I felt he knew it by the way he constantly preened his hair. There was no doubt in my mind that he knew he could have any woman he wanted, so I kept questioning why I didn't see a ring on his wedding finger. *He must be gay; that must be it,* I thought to myself as he talked on about sanitation fluids as if it was the most interesting subject in the world.

In the early days, I found working for Peter irritating. He was a perfectionist and never let anything slide. It drove me crazy. He would keep me sitting in front of him for what seemed an eternity while I waited for one of his long lectures to end so I could get back to work. He was forcing me to look at him, and I hated that. I went to great lengths to avoid him, certain that he thought I liked him, which simply wasn't true.

As time went on, I got to know Peter's humorous side and found myself, against my own will of course, liking him very much. I found he was actually quite modest and unassuming, and also very patient and kind. He was willing to take the time to explain something I should have understood – like expressing cubic dimensions. I was able to predict his comments and expectations, always one step ahead of him, and I took pleasure in seeing his satisfaction at a job done well. We were so in tune with each other, there were weeks we both wore the same coloured tailored shirts every day without even trying.

One evening the Commercial Director and I sat at our kitchen table drinking wine. I kept talking about work and Peter, 'God, it's like he's an old grandmother. He picks everything to pieces. He's so irritating!' I said.

'Really? What do you mean?'

'I mean I have to get more than five quotes before I can appoint a printer. He makes me sit in front of his desk whilst he corrects my press releases like a schoolteacher. He takes forever to make decisions and get on with things. He's just so…. Oh, I don't know. He just bugs me.'

Commercial Director poured me more wine and I continued

complaining about how much my boss irritated and drove me crazy. Then suddenly something dawned on me. If he bugged me so much, why had I just spent my entire evening talking about him? Before I even thought about what I going to say, I blurted out 'Oh my God. I think I've fallen in love with him!' Not the kind of love I had known up to this point, but the kind of love I dreamed of as a little girl. Peter made me forget to breathe when he was near. He gave me butterflies and I felt like I had jumped from a hundred-story building and was free falling completely out of control. It wasn't just about the nice falling in love feelings. I had grown to trust Peter too; he was kind and considerate, a real stand up kind of man – unlike Commercial Director who had hurt me several times by fooling around with other women. When Peter smiled at me, I felt warm and sweet inside like sticky toffee pudding. As I went into great depth explaining my feelings about another man to the Commercial Director, he poured the rest of my wine down the sink and told me to go to bed.

I staggered up to our room and fell into bed already half asleep. The following morning I had forgotten what I said, but very quickly recalled when Commercial Director recoiled when I tried to wrap my arm around him. The conversation came flooding back and I apologised profusely. I even told him I'd quit my job if he wanted me to, but he said, 'No. I'm willing to share you.' WHAT? This was the answer of a man who couldn't keep his jolly Rodger in his pants for more than a few minutes. Was I meant to share too? I was given an ultimatum: I could marry him and have a secure home for my son, or I could leave and possibly end up on my own with no money, no home, and no prospects. Putting my son's needs before my own, I made the decision to marry.

Within six months, I knew I couldn't pretend anymore. I wanted out. Commercial Director asked me to go on one last holiday with him to work through my feelings before taking such a drastic step. We went to Madeira. After a couple of days my birth control pills were suddenly nowhere to be found. On the fifth night, Commercial Director tried to sexually force himself on me. I clawed at his face as he held his hand over my mouth so I couldn't scream. There wasn't much chance of me getting away from him, so I was very lucky that he decided to let me go. I immediately packed my bags, went to the hotel lobby and asked them to order me a taxi.

Not knowing where else to go, I was dropped off at the airport at 2 AM. I sat on the floor with my suitcase next to me. I leaned against a wall and heavily sighed wondering what to do next. There was no one around to help and I was tired. I decided to ring Peter and tell him what happened. He kindly ordered a taxi to pick me up and take me to a hotel to spend the night. He also arranged a flight home for me the next day. After a restless sleep, I caught my flight and Peter collected me from the airport. He had booked a room for me that evening at the luxurious Ashdown Park Hotel. He wanted to give me some time to consider the way forward. That night we had dinner at the hotel and talked. I was so nervous and stressed that I was quite visibly drenched in sweat and had to go to my room to change.

The following day I went home to collect some personal belongings and proceeded to check myself into a hotel local to my work. PJ was with James at the time, so I had some explaining to do when I collected him. Fortunately, he was young enough to take it in his stride, or so I tried to convince myself. We settled into the hotel for a couple of months during which time Peter and I started dating.

Chapter 31

Peter

It was 1999, and I moved again to another place – this time it was with Peter.

I had finally completed my Marketing Degree and was quickly promoted to Marketing Manager. I continued to work in that capacity for a year before resigning. Perhaps it was because I was female, or because I obviously got on well with the boss, but the other staff members were difficult with me, lacking in support towards me both professionally and personally. This created many problems for me executing my responsibilities. Following my resignation, Peter and his father Myles called a meeting to see if they could smooth over the rough edges and retain my services.

Peter began, 'I guess the whole point of this meeting is to ask if you really want to resign or if we can come to an agreement.'

I said that obviously it would be easier to stay – I had put my heart into my job and would like to make it work.

'What we'd really like to know is if you will ever really be happy here, or will this keep happening?'

'Yes, I think if I had more support from the staff I could be much happier.'

Myles, who really wanted me to go, chimed in, 'You're no more important than anybody else. If everybody has a problem with you maybe you should look to yourself.'

'I really resent your implication. Look, I didn't ask for this meeting.'

'All I'm saying is maybe you're the one with the problem.'

I was being attacked, so true to my fighting nature, I stood up and walked out of the meeting, and as I did I couldn't help mutter under my breath, 'Assholes.'

Things weren't going well. Myles didn't know Peter and I were dating, and this episode was not going to make telling him any easier.

The next morning I ate a huge piece of humble pie by going into Myles' office to apologise for my hot temper. I explained that he was very hurtful in what he had said and I felt provoked. However, I was still very sorry for disrespecting him in that way. He said it was Peter I should be apologising to. Maybe he knew more than he was letting on.

Peter and I dated for nearly two years before he told his family about me. This became a real cause of disagreement between his family and us. I felt I was the one they didn't approve of, the American girl who had called Daddy an asshole. Peter hadn't involved them from the start, and I believe they were very angry and annoyed with not having any input. Unfortunately their anger was directed at me, even though I begged Peter to tell them from the beginning. Peter had decided that with the way things stood between his father and me, and his situation in the family business, that it was unwise to rock the boat. I felt very dirty during that time, as if Peter was ashamed of me.

After Peter told his family about us, his father said many hurtful things. Things that implied I only wanted Peter's money and that I was a hard, calculating woman who needed an eye kept on. His family talked about me as if I was a dirty rag that nobody knew what to do with. I know all of this because Peter told me. With so much negative attention directed at me, I felt everything I did was under scrutiny. At times the pressure to perform was too much to bear. As a result, once again I retreated deep inside and they demanded to know why I was so unsocial and not making an effort.

Terribly upset by a conversation Peter's father had with another family member, I called Peter's mother in tears one day looking for warmth and understanding. What I got was, 'What did you expect? With your past and everything that you've been through, of course there's bound to be talking. It's only natural we would have our concerns and reservations.' I hung up the phone not knowing how to feel. Just because I had a rocky life didn't make me any less of a caring and beautiful woman.

Nevertheless, what did I expect? Did I really believe a family, who on the surface had it all, would take me into their comfortable inner circle with no questions asked? Then I thought, *'but if Peter loves me for who I am, surely this is enough for them. Surely they have enough faith in his judgement to give me the benefit of the doubt.'* It frightened me to think that I would never be respected for the person I am. I would always be fighting an invisible demon – expected to seek their approval if I wanted to be accepted and part of the family. This thought alone made me want to give up before I even began.

Slowly the situation became more tolerable but has never been effortless between his family and me. They didn't and don't understand why I'm so quiet, and I didn't and don't understand why it is so important for me to be gregarious and not myself towards them.

Chapter 32

A final abandonment

On a chilly October day, nearly a year after Peter and I moved in together, I received a call from Sheila telling me Terry was in the hospital dying from cancer. Having left PJ with James' mum, two days later I was on a plane travelling towards Clearwater, Florida to see my dying ex-mother.

I hadn't seen Terry in 10 years and was deeply shocked at the state of her. She was drawn and emaciated, looking more like a 75 year old than the 52 she was. I went to her side and my hands shook as I touched hers. I couldn't stop my tears from flowing freely. 'Hi Mommy.'

'Hey Tiger.'

'God, you look like shit.'

'At least I don't have to worry about my weight now.'

While a nurse came in and topped up Terry's painkillers I thought, *she's abandoning me again, as if the first time didn't hurt enough. Not only that, but she's doing it without any remorse or explanation about the past.*

It's very difficult to remain angry with a person who is suffering so much pain; surely this was payment enough for all her faults. I told her I forgave her, even though she acted like there was nothing to forgive. I felt like our roles had reversed. She was the defiant, insolent child and I was the patient parent.

I sat down next to her as she lay in her hospital bed struggling to breath, and after a while of listening to her gasp for air, I asked, 'What kind of fish was that?' She sparked into life like she did the day we were on the hump back bridge. Eyes wide with excitement she said, 'That bad boy was a Pike!' I told her we shouldn't have been fishing there; the sign said so. She quickly reminded me of the pact we had made that day, saying that the sign was on the other side of the bridge facing away so we couldn't see it... 'Remember?' Oh, of course. Then she said, 'Do you remember that day I got you stoned? You were so cute.'

'You weren't supposed to do things like that. I was only a child.'

'Yeah, you were so beautiful.'

I leaned over and laid my head down on her bed holding her hand. We both shut our eyes and remained silent for over half an hour. I recalled a time when I was 5 when we pulled up to a 7 – 11 convenience store in Massachusetts. She asked me to jump out and get her a bag of ice from the outdoor freezer. I refused, saying she'd only steal it. She promised me she wouldn't. I had her word. Being the obedient daughter, I went and got the ice. She placed it on the seat next to her while I climbed into the back of the car. She hit the accelerator and sped away without paying. She laughed, but I didn't. Why couldn't she just be honest? Why wouldn't she do the right thing just once in her life?

Suddenly Terry's voice roused me from my deep thoughts and I was back in the hospital room again. She said, 'That was a nice walk. Thank you.' Once again my tears began to fall. She then asked me to please leave.

The next day I went to see Terry and the first thing out of her mouth when she saw me was, 'I don't have any money you know. So, if that's what you're here for you've got another think coming.'

'I'm not here for money. You're dying. That's why I'm here.' I said rolling my eyes in disbelief.

There was a long silence, and I went to her side and sat down. Suddenly she said, 'When I get out of this joint I'm going back to Texas. I love that place.' It seemed pointless to remind her again that she was dying. Even in her deathbed she was still planning to run away just as she always had throughout her life. Every time things got difficult, she moved homes and entire states. This time it was back to Texas.

Later that day, the doctors discharged her to her sister Anita who would be giving her hospice care in her trailer. Terry was in so much pain she could hardly move. We made it to Anita's and within a couple of hours had to take Terry back to the hospital because she needed stronger pain control and more radiotherapy.

Her poor body was riddled with cancer – there wasn't one bit of her that didn't ache.

On the way out of Anita's, there was a very small step and Terry was terrified of the pain it was going to cause her. She cried like a little girl, 'I'm scared. I'm so scared.' I tried to reassure her it would be OK as we dragged her down despite her screams of pain. I couldn't bear it. I sobbed all the way back to the hospital which was half an hour away.

When Sheila arrived from North Carolina we were just returning from Anita's and met her outside Emergency. She looked at me and then at Terry. When she saw the state Terry was in, you could see the pain of grief strike her as if somebody had just clenched her heart in his fist. Her eyes looked like she had seen something her brain couldn't comprehend. Sheila's a tough woman, but she couldn't fool me. We hugged and cried together.

Tina chose not to go to Florida to say goodbye, and I can't say I blame her. She was currently clean and sober and something like this would have sent her over the edge again. To be fair, I don't even know why I was there.

On the third day of my visit, Sheila and I both went to see Terry in hospital. She had received more pain medication and radiotherapy and was in better spirits. When we arrived, she called me a 'sissy' for wearing a 'sissy dress' even before saying hello. Despite my anger that she could be so callous, both Sheila and I sat next to her each on either side holding her hand. Despite her shortcomings, we were loyal to the end. I have asked myself repeatedly why I was so forgiving, and the only answer I can come up with is because I am a beautiful person. There must be something good about her to have been able to create me. I have to believe that so I don't look in the mirror every day and hate myself.

Later that day, even though there was a Grade 4 hurricane blowing outside, Sheila and I left the safety of our beachfront motel and went for an exhilarating walk along the beach. The waves were ferocious throwing up beautiful seashells and creatures. The wind was heavy with precipitation and salt, leaving stickiness all over us. We had to lean into the gale to walk forward, vulnerable and exposed, but God did I feel so alive! As darkness enveloped us, Sheila and I sat on the beach. Feeling like a little girl going through the pain and separation of her mother,

I collapsed into Sheila's lap in tears. Sheila said nothing, just rubbed my back as I let go of a childhood of pain.

Within a couple of days, we moved Terry back to Anita's trailer. During one of our visits Uncle Dick came to see Mom. There was no warm, heartfelt hello between him and me. Terry said to him, 'Hasn't she changed!' He nodded his fat face and tacky dyed Elvis hair do up and down. I thought, *Yes haven't I? I am no longer the petite naïve blond girl who let you repeatedly whip her with a switch. Now I know the difference between right and wrong, and how to fight for justice. You come near me now, and I'll kick your family jewels up your back passage!* I nodded back at him smiling sweetly as I imagined doing so.

Uncle Dick didn't come near, nor did he apologise for hurting me so much when I was a little girl. He didn't ask me how I was, or if I had a family. He asked me if I had some British money, and I did, so I showed him. That was the extent of our conversation because I didn't ask him about his family either. In retrospect, at least we were honest – neither of us making more of the situation than it was. Uncle Dick and I were near strangers forced to talk again because we had a common bond; Terry was his sister and she was my ex-mother.

When Sheila and I had to leave a few days later, we stopped by Anita's trailer to see Terry. She was lying in bed and I went to her side to say a final goodbye. 'I love you Lora Lee.' It was the first time during my stay that she had used my real name. I wondered if she really knew what love is. Not knowing what else to say, I told her I loved her too – questioning my meaning of the words as well. When it was time to go, I stood at the door, twisting the handle ready to leave. I turned and held her eyes trying to speak volumes without saying a word. She knew she would never see me again. I knew there would never be any answers, and that I would never again see the woman who gave birth to me. It took everything in me to turn around and leave, shutting the door gently behind me. Having already returned my rental car, I climbed into Sheila's pickup truck and we drove away slowly and carefully, almost as if we might break. We were both silent. I was thinking, *'No more tears, no more hurting. No more lies, one final abandonment.'* We drove on feeling a sense of closure at last.

When I returned home I received an email from Terry, the last piece of correspondence I was to have from her:

Wednesday, 4th October 2000, 11:16 AM, 'You have asked for me to try and sort of weed out your life as best I could. Where do I begin Lora Lee? You've asked who your father is and as always I've told you, George Hampton Bradley is, but that Larry Lee Ketler signed the paternity papers at the hospital to avoid any hassle or bull from George. Larry was a very good man and had all intention on raising you also Sheila and Tina as his own. I have had contact with him and his wife with which I believe we've discussed (we hadn't). Because of Tina's mind trips is where I started getting upset again. Doesn't she realise how many lives she has destroyed and tried to ruin through her lies? I need to stop for now. This is where I get all afloat in feelings. It's hard to keep things straight in my mind. What is left of it anyway. I was really thinking of just using the small tape recorder I had to rattle this into. I know there is a lot of different info you've gotten. Before I go any further, did you ever get a hold of Larry or Martha Ketler? Or did you get caught up with all the riff raff Ms Tina was flinging around at the Moment. I really can't remember. I use to keep records as to the attacks. But I believe I got ticked and threw away a whole bunch of papers and decided I wasn't going to dwell on the past Bull which 9 times out of 10 was exactly all that!! I know and realise I could *have picked a lot of different ways to get away from your father but at my age, your father's rank, the dear blessed golden years era, being the unforgivable Catholic church. If you weren't married, etc, etc... but for a mere $10 thousand dollars the church would recognise you back into their click. I'm having Anita type this much up and maybe we can chip the pieces we are looking for. Here is the info on Larry. (Withheld for sake of privacy). He is a telephone operator in Kansas. Maybe he could help you out on a watts line. I know he would love hearing from you. I believe I told Sheila also, but feel I got a block there also. Maybe not. But I'm sure you've got the mother's intuition feeling before. Let's give this a stab between us. That's it for now. I love you, Momsy.'*

There were no more emails from Terry, and I sent one final email to her on the 9th November that simply read, *'Goodbye Mommy. I love you. Be a good girl.'*

The next day I received a phone call to tell me she was dead. Again. It was strange, I don't know how I knew her time was up, but I did. I felt it in my soul. I didn't cry, I had already said my good-byes. The act was now final and I recalled her words to me in the hospital when I sat by her side, 'Life moves on Tiger.' And so it did.

A couple of weeks later I received a large package from Florida. In it I found Terry's watch amongst other things. I held it watching the second hand tick – thinking about life moving on. I sifted through numerous photos of what was going to be my family. There were photographs of people who were going to be Cousins, Aunties, Uncles, Grand Parents, and Great Grandparents. There were numerous photos of her with her brother and two older sisters, and old black and white shots of her on the knee of her grandfather. The only photos I did not see were with her daughters. In fact, I realised that one of the only photographs I had ever seen of us together, mother and daughter, was the one Sheila took in the hospital before she died.

I was surprised to find a family tree dating back to September 1668 showing my ancestors on my grandmother's side were from Normandy, France. I discovered not only that, but there are also priests and nuns in what was going to be my family. There's one photo of Terry around ten years old dressed in white, going through catechism.

How can one woman cause so much damage to a family tree? My sisters and I will be the chink in the chain for generations to come. I thought to myself, *I will make a difference and reunite the family line. I don't want to be the embarrassing part of my biological family's history. I want to be the one that did something special and wonderful with her life despite the odds.* The idea really inspired me and I hugged it to myself.

Amongst the other artefacts in the package, I found a video. I stuck it into the machine and hit PLAY. It was a family Christmas celebration. The people who were going to be my family were unwrapping presents and laughing. Terry was drunk wobbling to and fro on her hands and knees on the kitchen floor as she tried to sop up her spilled drink. She was heavily slurring her words, but nobody seemed to even notice her. They stepped around and talked over her. Why? Why didn't any of these people who were supposed to be my family ever come for me? Why didn't they ask about me, care about me, and want us three girls in their family? Why would they send me a video like this and why would I never hear from 'Aunt Anita' or 'Uncle Dick' again after Terry died?

In the package there were also some newspaper clippings. One main headline on the front page of the Ayer Free Press on

Wednesday, December 18, 1963, Littleton, Massachusetts read, 'Littleton Girl Seriously Injured in Auto Accident,' and the sub headline read, 'Three Others Taken To Hospital After Car Hits Tree on Harwood Ave.' The next clip appeared on the front page of The Littleton Independent on Tuesday, December 31, 1963. 'Marsha Wallace Showing Improvement in Hospital,' and the sub-headline read, 'Injured Girl Speaks for First Time since Dec. 13.' The Littleton girl they are referring to is Terry. She changed her name from Marsha Anne to Terry Jean later in life.

In 'The Anatomy of Hope' by Dr Jerome Groopman, I read about the tale of Phineas Gage, a railroad foreman who suffered a freakish accident in the summer of 1848. While he was overseeing a laying of track, a metal spike flew up and penetrated Gage's skull, just behind his forehead. Remarkably, the spike passed into the frontal lobes of the brain but didn't kill him. Furthermore, when it was removed, Gage woke up from his coma. Initially, it was difficult to discern the effects of the damage on his brain, but they became clear from his behaviour. The injury left him emotionally bereft as well as devoid of the capacity to reason. In the ensuing years, other patients who had parts of their frontal lobes damaged or removed because of trauma, tumours, or a psychiatric treatment were found to resemble Gage. Their emotions were shallow, and they suffered deficits in deliberate reasoning.

Terry had hit the front of her head hard as she flew through the windscreen and landed against a tree. There is every probability the impact caused damage to her frontal lobes. Maybe that's why she made such a mess of her life. I keep looking for reasons, and more came when in an attempt to piece together some of the unexplained, I wrote an email to Terry's sister Anita. I was taken aback at the tone of reply and have included them in example of what my sisters and I are treated like by our biological family:

Subject: *Are you still on this address?*
To: *Anita*

I'm so pleased I am able to get in touch with you still. I am currently writing an autobiography but I have so many questions about Terry that I was hoping you could help me with. Like, is it true she had a baby before Tina was born that died in her crib? And was she locked in the basement of Pepe's when she had Tina until they could find her a husband? Personally, why do you think she went off the rails so spectacularly? Was she different after her car accident? Is there anything you can remember about her that you'd like to share? I want to paint a fair and accurate picture of her upbringing. Can you help me?

By the way, are you still dating the same bloke? How is Richard (Uncle Dick)? Is he still having problems with his back?

Really so pleased to hear from you after so long, and hope you are able to help me.

Lots of love, Lora Lee x

Reply received three weeks later:

I just got back on line again. To answer your questions:

1- No, your mother didn't have a baby before Tina.
2- No, she wasn't locked in basement until she found a husband. She married Wally who had gotten her pregnant.
3- She changed after her car accident. After all she was in a coma for 3 months.

I don't remember that much because I was out of the house & married, sorry.

No, I wasn't going with anybody special at that time. Dick is hoping to have back surgery this coming Thursday if the heart doctor says it's ok.

Anita

Reply email from me sent the next day:

Hi Anita,

Tina wanted to know who Wally is. She's confused by the newspaper article about Terry being in hospital because it says she's married to Bob Wallace, and that they had a daughter together in 1963. Tina's father was John Wallace and she was born in 1965... When we were little Terry used to say she had a little girl named Maryann who died a crib death.

Sheila has said that we have American Indian in our family. Is this something you can clarify for me?

I'm sorry to ask, but you are one of the only people left who can help us piece together our fragmented lives. We want to get the story right for our children.

Thank you,
Lora Lee

Reply from Anita the following day:

Wally was the nickname for John Wallace. Maryann was our sister, not Marsha's (Terry's) daughter.

Yes, we are of a Canadian Indian Tribe not American, but I don't know the name of them. If I find out I will let you know.

Marsha (Terry) made her First Communion on May 26th, 1956. Confirmation on May 16th, 1961. Anita

Final email sent by me the same day:

Hi Anita,

Sorry to bother you again. I've just re-read the newspaper article that Tina was on about, and it quite clearly says that her (Terry's) husband Bob was fighting in Korea, that they had been married for a year by that point (13th Dec 1963) and had one child together. If she didn't have another baby, what on earth are they talking about... and who is Bob? Is it possible Terry did have another baby and because you were living away in your married home didn't know? We are just so confused – especially considering Terry always told us Maryann was her baby. One thing is certain – they aren't talking about Tina because Tina was born in Feb 1965. Any ideas? Lora Lee x

I never had a reply, and am still none the wiser. One thing is for certain: Terry was raised in an extremely Catholic family that would obviously go to great lengths to remain an upstanding family in their religious circle. Tina, Sheila and I are obvious ink splotches on a pristine family tree. We are not recognised by our own family, and even the baby Maryann that died a crib death lays in an unmarked grave in Fitzburg, Massachusetts nobody wanting to take responsibility for her life and death. The more I delve into Terry's past, the more I discover, and her story remains to be told another day.

Chapter 33

Sister Kay

About a year after Terry's death, I received an email from Mom and Dad saying my sister Kay had an enormous lump on her leg – just where mine had been. At first the doctors said it was a cyst, but Mom insisted they take further tests. Unfortunately, the further tests revealed it was Sinovial Cell Cancer. This type of cancer is generally quite treatable, but Kay had waited so long to seek medical treatment the tumour on her leg was the size of a grapefruit. Consequently she had minimal response to chemotherapy, and radiotherapy was cut short because the treatment had left her with second-degree burns. Following the initial unsuccessful treatments, surgery was performed to remove the tumour from her leg and stop it spreading elsewhere in her body.

The removal of the tumour left Kay with a drop foot and she had to wear a leg brace to walk; other than that, all seemed fine. A couple of months later I received a call from Mom. She started, 'She didn't tell us the news at first, and the doctors weren't allowed to tell us because technically she is an adult, but I knew something was wrong and I insisted she tell me.'

'What are you saying, Mom?'

'The cancer has spread to her lungs.'

'Mom, that's serious isn't it? I mean, don't people usually die once it has spread to their lungs?' Mom said that was the case very matter-of-factly, and I was left stunned. She said they were looking to see if any new medical trials would accept Kay, and if there weren't, the next option was trying a different kind of chemotherapy.

There were no medical trials and Kay's chemotherapy was once again unresponsive, so the doctors suggested surgery to physically remove the one tumour they could clearly see on her lungs.

I flew out to the States for a couple of weeks to be with my family during her operation and recovery. The morning of Kay's surgery, as we all waited for her name to be called at the San Francisco Medical Centre, I felt certain the outcome was not going to be good, but kept this depressing thought to myself and held back my tears.

Following surgery Mom, Dad and I waited anxiously in her room for the results. The surgeon came in and calmly explained that once he had gone in, he didn't find just one tumour but lungs full of them. He had removed as much as he could without compromising her ability to survive and sewn her back up. He said she could continue to have the same major surgery every six months to remove the lumps that would continue to grow, and this could extend her life for a while, but he couldn't say how long a while was.

My dear brave 20-year-old sister made the decision she didn't want any further medical intervention. She was going to make the most of her final days and enjoy them instead of suffering through medical treatment and then dying. Such a huge decision for someone so young, but she was adamant that's how her disease was to run its course.

The rest of my family obviously had their strong beliefs about what Kay should do, but as Kay was 'officially an adult', and even though she didn't act like one most of the time, she had the final say. As her sister and being very close to her, it was very difficult to stand back and watch her waste away. She was vastly overweight and continued to eat only ice cream and sugary snacks instead of trying to prolong her life by eating healthy foods to stimulate her body's ability to fight. Being a cancer survivor, I was shocked at her willingness to die. I struggled with the fact that she seemed to have no fight in her. I wondered if she wanted to die. Was she taking the easy route out, or did she have a quiet resolve — a sixth sense that told her it was her time and to accept it gracefully?

Hearing the news that my little sister was going to die (not may die, but 100% definitely would die and probably soon), started me thinking about my own mortality and brushes with death, and how I handled that threat compared to Kay. When I tried to explain to Kay how bad I felt at her predicament, she told me our parents said I felt guilty that I survived my cancer and she wouldn't. I explained to her that I never for one moment felt guilty that I survived my cancer. What I did feel guilty about was my ability to handle my situation with so much more fight, determination, and inner strength than she could ever muster. I felt like I was watching a fowl trying to find her legs, but her every attempt to stand and be strong kept failing. She was simply giving up and accepting her destiny, her legs buckled under her waiting for a predator to finish the job. While Kay was the proverbial lamb, I was the intrepid fox who would have gnawed my own leg off if it meant the freedom to live and see another day. I felt guilty that I had this ability and she did not. It may not be the most endearing, ladylike trait but it kept me alive and I wished that much for her.

After Kay's devastating news, Mom, Dad, Kay and brother Will came to visit for the first time since I moved to England through the *Make a Wish* charity that generously grants terminally ill children one last wish. Kay wanted to visit me. Now, if she had known she could have met her favourite football player instead, no doubt she would have changed her mind! Kay had a thing for men wearing tight spandex and throwing a ball. As it was, *Make a Wish* paid for the first class flights, gave our parents spending money to pay for all meals and taxi rides, paid for a private cubicle on the London Eye and a day of sight seeing in London. If that wasn't enough they also arranged a make-over for us ladies in a top London department store, gave us tickets to go see *The Lion King* in the West End, and arranged a limousine to pick us up from our hotel and take us shopping at Harrods followed by tea at the Ritz. Kay was still able to walk on her own, and the painkillers she took to ease the pain of the growing masses in her lungs remained manageable, so we were able to keep up with the exhausting schedule and have a wonderful time.

One memory that stands out in my mind was our shopping trip to Harrods. Mom, Dad and Will went one direction while Kay and I went another. Kay was a Tomboy, so she wanted to go and look at the store's collection of baseball caps. When we had finished looking, she asked me to hold the bag she was carrying saying she was tired. I could understand that; we had been on our feet all day, and with her being so overweight, it didn't surprise me she was finding it difficult.

At the designated time, we met our parents and Will and proceeded to pile into the waiting limousine. As we drove along to our next destination, Mom wanted to see what Kay had bought, so she started pulling merchandise out of the bag I had just been carrying. The first thing she pulled out was a baseball cap that Kay didn't pay for, but I was the only person besides Kay that knew that. I immediately flashed my knowing and accusing eyes at Kay, and she held my stare defiantly as if to say it was her right to steal – she was going to die. Although I couldn't for the life of me understand why she felt the need to steal anything with parents and an adoring older sister who would have happily paid for anything she wanted, I found I could still forgive her. What I couldn't forgive was her asking me to carry the bag with the stolen cap out of the store. What if alarms had sounded? Would she have also allowed me to be arrested in her place? Kay's disturbed behaviour had me in a continual state of flux between wanting to mother her and wanting to strangle her for her childish behaviour. She had always been like that – I don't know why I had presumed having cancer would change her.

If I felt completely used up by Kay's trying behaviour as her older sister who only had to deal with her at arm's length, imagine how my parents felt who had to live with her on a daily basis. If it wasn't one thing, it was another. For instance, the time she was caught packing a loaded gun at school. When my parents asked her how she had come to have a loaded gun, she said that a friend had asked her to hold it for him. What made it most bizarre is that she was a genuinely loving and intuitive young woman that could charm the green off a leprechaun. She was tormented by her own mental instability, laughing uncontrollably one moment and crying for no reason the next. We all accepted and understood this about Kay, but it didn't make it easier to handle. People who didn't know our family well, and sometimes the odd cruel family member that did, would inevitably look to my parents and wonder what they had done to cause Kay to behave in such a manner. In my parent's defence, I have to say my poor parents did the best they could with such a needy and challenging young woman.

Kay stayed with me an extra week following my family's departure because she wanted to go to Paris. Despite the fact that I was due to open my new business, Happy Days (an out of school activity club for 4 to 13 year olds) and could have used the few short days left before opening my doors to get my staff and myself prepared, I decided to spend the time with my sister because that was what she wanted. Everything else just had to wait.

In our hotel room in Paris, Kay said 'Sissy?'

'Yep?' I called out from the bathroom as I unpacked my toiletries.

'I'm feeling really tired now. Can we stay in for a bit?'

'Yes, of course. I'll just have a bath while you rest.'

As I enjoyed the Jacuzzi bath I began to hear strange noises in the other room. 'What is that, Kay?' I shouted to her. I heard Kay laughing and more odd groaning noises. I got out of the tub, wrapped a towel around me and went to find Kay lying on the bed watching a porno. 'KAY! I'm telling Mom!' She didn't say anything. She just lay there with a mischievous grin on her face watching the TV. I had never seen a pornographic movie before, so I sat on the bed next to her and watched. 'Oh my God… that's disgusting. Ewww!'

'Yuck what is that on his dick?' Kay said completely grossed out.

'You don't know what that is? It's foreskin. Haven't you ever seen foreskin before?'

'Ewww – no – yuck.'

I watched some more and laughed at the bad acting. 'Something must be wrong with his balls because they won't show them. Oh look, see! They're really small!' I said. 'OK, if you had to rate his willy between 1 – 10, 10 being the best, what would you give him?'

'It's not very big and it has foreskin, so I don't rate him at all.'

'Hmmm… it's not that bad, but his small balls ruin it for me. I'd give him a two.' I said.

'I'm telling Peter you watched a porno!'

'Don't you bloody dare' I said throwing a pillow at her.

We enjoyed our special four summer days in Paris going to all the usual tourist destinations, which involved a great deal of walking; something Kay didn't do a lot of. The memories we made far outweigh many others we shared together as sisters. She was so jovial. I made her into a video queen, taping her every move, and of course she made me into a porn queen!

When it came time to check out, Kay made me pay for the porn separately from the main bill in case Mom was to see the bill. I felt my face burning as I explained to the front desk what I wanted to do. Kay thought it was wonderful to see her older sister dying of embarrassment.

When we returned from Paris, Kay left the next morning for home. I couldn't stop sobbing as I watched her escorted through to the departure lounge. The fear I would not see her ever again seized my heart as I watched her disappear.

Chapter 34

Tink

Over a year later, now 2003, I gave birth to Peter's and my first child together, Thomas Myles (Tink).

I must have forgotten how difficult and painful childbirth was because I decided to have a water birth. I was writhing in pain shouting that I wanted painkillers and an epidural, and I wanted them NOW! The midwife said there was no time to give me any pain relief – my baby was coming too quickly. I shouted at her, 'HOW DO YOU KNOW?' splashing her face as my angry fist came down and hit the water. She replied very determinedly, 'because I have been doing this for 23 years. Now BREATHE!'

I was only in the hospital a day following Tink's birth before I had to rush home. By then Happy Days was in full swing and none of my employees knew how to drive such a large manual vehicle, so I had to pick up from several local schools a mini bus full of screaming children.

Although I started Happy Days hopeful it would help me forge new friendships with other ladies my age, it turned out most of the mothers resented me, and Happy Days ended up being the unhappiest days of my life. The logistics involved in picking up 32 children after school and delivering them to our premises where we entertained them until their parents arrived by 6:30 pm were simply a nightmare. During summer it was an all day affair from 7 am – 6:30 pm, which was incredibly exhausting. The stress of meeting the strict OFSTED regulations, staff continually letting me down, dealing with dishonest parents who resented paying their bills, and having to tote Tink with me everywhere I went and worry for his safety, all proved simply too much to handle in the end. After three and a half years of operating, I shut Happy Days down with a great sense of relief.

Chapter 35

Saying goodbye

Around 4 pm on a warm summer's day, Peter answered the telephone. I was upstairs changing Tink's nappy when he appeared with the phone. An intensely sad expression etched into his face told me I wasn't going to like what I was about to hear. I took the phone and said 'hello?' in a mere whisper.

It was Dad. He was crying. My little sister, age 21, had just passed away. He tried to give details, but was too upset and handed the phone to Mom. I told Mom how sorry I was. 'I can't believe she died on your birthday.' I couldn't think of what else to say – there's not a lot one can say to ease the pain of losing a child. We were both in a muddle of emotions.

I hung up the phone and stood frozen on the landing staring down our hall. Like ghosts before me, I suddenly saw Sheila with the palm of her hand pressed on the back window of the car being driven away from me. I saw my biological mother just before I said good-bye and shut the door. I saw the woman in the funeral home laying in a peaceful permanent rest. I felt my own mortality as I saw myself lying in a hospital bed receiving chemotherapy. I felt the pain I felt when my mother never came back for me. I relived the ache I felt as I saw my little sister escorted away from me at the airport. I felt and saw so much pain I couldn't stand. I reached for something to steady me as I fell to my knees in agony. I wanted to scream, 'It's not fair! I am hurting so much. Why me? Why her? WHY?' Instead, I just held my face in my hands unable to face the truth, trying to rock myself into a state of numbness.

No matter how much you try to prepare yourself for what you know is bound to happen, it still comes as a shock. Perhaps it's the finality of it. Knowing that there are no more chances to say, 'I love you,' or 'I'm sorry.' Knowing that whatever memories you had with them – that's it, no more can be made or experienced. Maybe it's the feeling of being powerless or knowing that I'll never see her grow older, get married and have babies. She will always be the tough, slightly disturbed 21-year old girl, and nothing I do can change that. Nothing can change the fact that she suffered a 2-½ year battle with cancer that eventually riddled her lungs and took her life.

I cried a lifetime worth of sorrow. I let the pain escape me in deep resounding sobs. I cried so hard, all the blood vessels around my eyes popped, but when I tired of crying I had no energy to stop and cried some more.

The day Kay died I had glimpsed all the pain I'd filed away, but the stronghold of thick walls and chilling numbness returned with even greater determination. I told myself I could handle whatever it was lurking just below my surface waiting to blow. I would not accept the past as my own or admit that I was the same person who had witnessed so many tragic events; therefore, I could not feel the pain that other girl and woman did. I could look at her feelings as if I was looking at a rat caught in a maze and sympathise but feel assured I was safe elsewhere. Without even realising it, I was slowly killing myself. I was choking any possible outlet for pain and expression not realising it had to come out somehow.

My parents held a memorial service at their church that was attended by many, but for whatever reason I wasn't invited. Instead, a year later my parents, brother Will, Peter, PJ, Tink and I chartered a boat in Half Moon Bay and scattered her ashes at sea. My biggest regret from that day is not hugging my brother when he cried after Kay's ashes were scattered. I should have made a point of reaching out and bonding with Will, but felt too distant from him emotionally to risk rejection.

Chapter 36

Being a mother

I gave birth to two more sons after Kay died – Giles Robert and Laurence Lee. My third son Giles was my smallest baby weighing in at 8 lbs 7 oz and became 'Jiggy' the day after he was born. To keep him quiet, I bounced him up and down saying, 'jiggy, jiggy, jiggy, jig' whilst doing it. Because he was a fussy baby, I used the word a lot, and the name suited him and stuck. He has always been Jiggy ever since, even though he keeps insisting I call him Giles today.

My fourth son Laurence Lee (named after me) was my heaviest boy weighing just a sliver shy of ten pounds. He is a calm, caring little person. The midwifes called him Bunny because he was born on Easter Sunday, but that was soon replaced by 'Lumpy Lou' because he continued to grow at an exponential rate being nearly as big as Jiggy by the age of two.

I love being a mother. It's what I am good at and what makes my life worthwhile. I have a strong sense of how to discipline and encourage my sons. I listen to my gut, draw on my ability to remember what I needed most from my mother as a child, and make sure I give it to my boys to the best of my ability. To me that means being affectionate, consistent, attentive, patient, happy, and strong. I show them I love them by caring enough to not only tickle and cuddle them, but also make them feel safe with clear boundaries and limits.

Do I see Terry in me? Of course I do. Alice once explained it all very clearly to me in her usual maternal way. She said I should remember all the great and wonderful things about Terry and add them to my personality, and take the rest of the horrible stuff, put it in a bag and throw it over a bridge. That's what I've tried to do as a mother and a person. Terry liked to sing and dance, create art, giggle, sit quietly and be still. These are all things I have added to myself in her memory. Besides liking my wine a little too much, sometimes I catch myself nearly back handing one of my sons in the same swift manner Terry used to, but stop myself short. At other times, I find myself staring across the room deep in thought and in a world of my own, and shake myself for alienating my children as Terry used to. I'm certainly not perfect, but I am aware of that and work hard every day to be the best mother I can be.

Mom, however, has had the most influence. She has been there for me consistently throughout the years, devoted to being my mother through thick and thin, showing me what true love is and how to express it in more than just words. She taught me it is OK to dislike my children sometimes, as long as I love them. I have learned from some of her mistakes too, and again have tried to make myself better in this way. For instance, Mom always busied herself to the point where she forgot to make time to kiss and cuddle me, or look at and appreciate a beautiful view. I too have the same tendency with my sons and forget to make down time for them. What I have learned most from both Mom and Dad is how to be a good role model for my own children, to admit when I have made a mistake and apologise, taking care not to make the same mistake again. In this way, I believe I am respecting my children as people, and in turn they will respect me too. That's the theory anyway!

Unlike my sister Sheila who raised her children with the full knowledge of all the horrific things we went through as children, I have not yet told my children about many aspects of my life mainly because I didn't want to remember memories long enough to explain them. I never wanted to burden them with the weight of my past sorrows. I wanted them, like everybody else, to know me for who I am now – not who I was then.

Yet I do wonder if they would have more respect for life and the woman I am if they knew the full extent of my past. PJ, my eldest son now 14 years old, knows I had a biological mother, but he has never asked why she didn't raise me or how I came to live with the Boyntons. He also knows I had cancer when I was younger, but he doesn't know what kind or the extent of the treatment and the likely outcome back then. He is comfortable and secure and doesn't question if I will be there for him in his future – he knows I will. He is trusting – just the way a child should feel. If I tell him that mothers leave their children in the middle of the night, or that he could be left as a result of illness, would his and my other sons' childhood and future seem a little less shiny?

Unfortunately I did reach a point where I realised that I was so into my children and being a good mother, I had forgotten to look after myself. Putting their every need before my own meant I had no energy left for me. I hadn't written, read, listened to music, walked, or sung in years, so I decided to start trying to do more things for myself. I began by writing Blogs on Myspace. It was a great way to reconnect with others and myself. In fact, I found Alice. I couldn't believe how beautiful and happy she looked. She has a husband, two children and is a reputable tattoo artist in Portland, Oregon. I sent her a message and we started up our friendship again. Writing on Myspace was a way to vent some of my pent up emotions and reach out not just to friends from the past, but to all sorts of people with similar worries or dilemmas.

BLOG – 'There, I said it...': *Driving along to drop my son off at nursery this morning, I started thinking about how much my life has changed since I came to England. Before the UK, I felt so vibrant, confident, at ease with myself. I had interests... I had a huge future before me. I think to myself 'maybe it's the English that have done this to me!' I get so tired of raised eyebrows and tight-lipped sneers when I say or do something decidedly American. Then it dawned on me, no what's really happened to change my life totally and completely was having children. I don't have time for myself anymore. I have to stay up until midnight or later if I want to chat online, or have a hot bath and read a book. My day is now filled with screaming, nappies, toys up to my ears, and good stuff too like giggles and hugs, but it's ALWAYS about them. I never get out on my own anymore. In fact, I feel painfully shy on my own and would much rather have my children with me. I pondered this for a while and then it hit me like a ton of bricks. I said to myself 'at least my children smile – therefore, I smile through them.'*

I thought of a conversation I had with some old friends whom we met up with in Sonoma on holiday last summer. I asked how they were; then how were their parents. My friend's husband said, 'God, you know, my mother really does need to stop trying to live her life through her children. She has no life of her own.'

'Hmmmm, yeah.... God that's terrible,' we all agreed. We would never do that. That's so selfish of her!

Now I'm sat here wondering if you can tell me how we are suppose to NOT live our lives through our children. How can we spend 20 years or more making their every need more important than our own and then suddenly one day rediscover ourselves; those past interests and youthful confidence a mere distant memory. I really want to know, because I don't want to wake up one morning and wonder who I am now that the last child has flown the nest. And let's admit it — they're all boys, which means it's worse: they don't look back often enough for mums, and don't have that sixth sense that mum may be down and need a telephone call, a bunch of flowers or to be taken to lunch like most women do for their mums from time to time. NOPE! My master plan needs to include a self-preservation clause to stop me from 'living my life through my children.'

My eldest son is a weekly boarder (by choice!) at a beautiful old school called Worth. When I went to pick him up for the weekend, I decided to take my new camera (part of my plan to keep my own interests) and walk with him. I proudly told the father of my 3 other children that I was going alone (with Laurence the baby of course), to spend some quality time with my eldest son and to have some time to myself.

'OK... OK... you go and have a good time.'

As I put my camera bag in the car, my second oldest son Tink started, 'want to go mummy' through thick tears. Grudgingly, I say "OK" get in. Then the one remaining son starts screaming and climbing the gate like a caged monkey.

'OOOHHHH! SCREW IT! GET IN!' So somehow what was suppose to be sometime to myself became Daddy's time. As we drove down the road, I wondered, 'How did he do that? Now I'm stuck with all the children again, and he's got the day off!'

So we get there, and it's a beautiful day. PJ was in good spirits and felt quite happy that I wanted to spend some time walking around the grounds of his school. I took loads of photos and let him take some too — showing him how to use the camera in simplest terms. We had a lovely time. The smaller boys enjoyed the natural playground of wooden stumps, throwing pebbles into the pond, climbing on anything and everything. I snapped loads of the children. God they are beautiful...

Looking back on the photos, I can see that for a brief moment I got the balance right; I was sharing my interests with my sons and also enjoying myself too. Not only that, I was teaching them new interests... Now I'm thinking, 'I can do this! It's tricky – this not living through your children stuff, but if I work at it maybe I won't lose myself in my boys anymore.' Except, in all honesty, taking the photos wouldn't have been as good as it was if they weren't there to make it such a pleasure.

Maybe I still need to work at it, but at least I recognise it and by saying it out loud, I have begun the path to my own life again.

Chapter 37

My demon

Following the birth of my fourth son Laurence Lee, I was struggling to breastfeed. I had tried everything. I even let the midwife try to express my milk because she was sure she could. She wasn't able to, and seemed a little shocked at how hard my nipple and breast was. In desperation, I went out and bought a breast milk expresser. That didn't work, so I bought an electric expresser. I tried laying in a hot bath and then expressing. Nothing. Not a drop. I had always had trouble breastfeeding, but nothing like this. Very worried and anxious, I set the electric pump to 'suck your nipple off' mode, and nothing came out but blood. All of this was torture when you consider I had mastitis. It was agonising. I had been on antibiotics a couple of times, but the mastitis always remained.

In one last attempt, whilst I massaged my nipple trying to soften it in hopes I would be able to miraculously express milk, I noticed a very small lump, about the size of a small pea, in the upper left hand quadrant of my nipple. There wasn't only a lump, but the skin retracted and the area around it was red, hot, and puffy. I recalled a conversation I had with Peter's sister where I asked her how she had known she had breast cancer. She said that she had seen a dimpling and sucking in of her skin.

Concerned, I went the next day to see my GP who fast tracked me to a consultant at a nearby hospital. I laid down while Mr 'I'm so wonderful' hastily examined my breast before telling me it was, 'probably just the remains of mastitis with some back flow obstruction of milk to the duct.' Probably. I was told not to worry, to continue breastfeeding if I wanted to, but that it wouldn't clear itself until I had stopped breastfeeding altogether.

I explained that this was my fourth child that I'd had mastitis before and this felt much different. Furthermore, I explained that I had cancer when I was young. He said in a flippant tone, 'Who knows why this has happened now.' He seemed in a hurry to get the observation and diagnosis over with. In fact, he was only in the room a total of three minutes.

Mr 'I'm so wonderful' wasn't in the least bit concerned by the fact that I had a history of mastitis that hadn't cleared after antibiotics. The fact that I had an inverted nipple, thickening, pain, and reddening of the skin did not ring alarm bells. Even though it is a known fact that if what appears to be an infection does not clear itself after a round of antibiotics, inflammatory breast cancer should not be ruled out, he still said it was nothing to worry about. Even though inflammatory breast cancer has a habit of presenting itself in women who are breastfeeding, he metaphorically tapped me on the head in a condescending manner and sent me on my way. He told me to come back seven weeks after I stopped breastfeeding, and strongly reassured me that there was nothing untoward occurring.

As Peter and I walked away, Mr 'I'm so wonderful' followed five steps behind with a colleague – presumably off to lunch, as it was that time of day. I said to Peter how arrogant I thought Mr 'I'm so wonderful' had been – that I was convinced something wasn't right. Peter said, 'Look darling, he's the expert; he does this for a living and knows what he's talking about. If he says it's a blocked milk duct, it must be a blocked milk duct.' That was that, and I chose to swallow it because it's what I wanted to believe.

A month later, I gave up breastfeeding on the other side. The redness and thickening of my skin had increased and looked like the skin of an orange and my nipple was even further retracted. As advised by Mr 'I'm so wonderful', I waited 7 weeks to see if the inflammation settled. It worsened and very quickly. My breast was double the size of my other.

When I rang to make an appointment, thinking 'Mr I'm so wonderful' would see me quickly, as there was obviously something untoward occurring, his secretary told me I would receive an appointment in the post. A week passed and I had heard nothing so I rang again. His secretary told me once again that an appointment would be arriving in the next couple of days. When the letter with my appointment did arrive, it suggested an appointment 3 months away. That was totally unacceptable! I contacted my GP, who contacted 'Mr I'm so wonderful's' secretary and requested the appointment be moved forward. It was by three weeks, except not with him but with a breast care nurse instead. Hearing this news, and feeling absolutely appalled by the lack of urgency, I decided to go privately because I KNEW whatever was happening inside my breast could not wait any longer.

Meanwhile, whilst all these worries about my breast floated around my head, I was also suffering from postnatal depression and was taking anti-depressants to try to level my anxieties. My depression and anxiety attacks became so severe I was frightened to leave the house. Some days I could barely tolerate dropping my sons off at nursery because it meant I would see people, and that may mean I would have to speak to them. I was in no fit state to hold a conversation. I couldn't even keep my own thoughts straight let alone articulate them. My hands shook when I tried to write, and my heart palpitated so fiercely I thought I was having a heart attack. The added worry over my health was soul destroying. I needed to see somebody fast to alleviate my fears before I went BANG!

In early August, I was referred to Mr Charles Zammit at the Nuffield Hospital, Brighton. Mr Zammit, originally from Malta, is very personable and humorous, so unlike the previous breast surgeon, I had an instant rapport with him.

He took his time going through my history leading up to the present. He then asked to examine my breasts. Upon inspection, he said he wanted to take a fine needle biopsy straight away. A little alarmed, I agreed – but told him I'm petrified of needles because of the cancer treatment I had when I was younger. He told me I forgot to mention I had cancer when he took my history, which I quite often do. I apologised sheepishly as the breast care nurse, Pam, came to my side and held my hand. She told Mr Zammit he had to the count of five to finish his task. My breast was very tender, and the needle hurt more than I expected it to.

'Owe!' I cried squeezing Pam's hand blue. It was taking Mr Zammit a lot longer than the count of five. He apologised saying he was finding it difficult to get the needle in where it needed to be. Finally he was finished, I went home, and the waiting began.

BLOG – 'My Demon'
My demon was coming for me. I could hear its heavy footsteps just around the corner and out of site. Panic was setting in. Every possible scenario played in my mind repeatedly to the point where I was giving myself a headache. It was my boyfriend's birthday, so we put on a brave face and went out to dinner under strict instructions not to discuss my breast in any shape or

form. *Why should we? Speculation is a waste of time at this stage. It could be nothing, so why worry? So, we made polite talk and had a pleasant meal and I struggled to refrain from talking about what was really on my mind. I hadn't had a drink in over 2 ½ months, but managed to drink a very intoxicating bottle of white wine which helped numb me a little. When we came home, I went up to my room and sat on the edge of my bed starring at the floor in deep thought for over an hour. Finally, I lied down and tried to sleep.*

After a very restless sleep, I spent the next day fidgeting, cleaning, reading and anything else I could think of to keep my mind off the pending telephone call. I felt panicky and driven to distraction. Luckily, my mother in law was here watching the boys, so I had a chance to isolate myself for a while. Finally, at 5:47 PM the phone rang. I was quite aware that the words he was about to speak could possibly change my life forever. Of course, things are never straightforward or simple, are they? He told me, 'We're going to take this in steps... (long pause). Most of your cells were benign' Most? What does that mean? He continued, 'There were, however, some cells that are worrying the pathologist. We need to take a larger tissue sample so we can study them more closely.'

Tunnel vision. Darkness sets in. He has spoken the words I was dreading to hear. My enormous dark demon is about to get me. I can't breathe, I can't move, I can't even protect myself or my family, and what's worse is that I can't even wake up from this fucking dream.

'I see, OK. Thank you then.' I hang up the phone. My whole world has changed. Yesterday it was just a fear,

and today it is a reality. Shocked and numb, I call my boyfriend then my mother. I need their opinion on what I just heard. What does it mean? How worried should I be?

That was two days ago. I go into the hospital this Wednesday for the deeper biopsy and ultra sound. We should know a lot more about what we are dealing with, but until then I've been fighting my demon non-stop trying to grab it by the horns and get a firm grip, but just when I think I've got control of the situation – that's the precise moment I lose my grip and everything threatens to overtake me – suffocate me. You see, this isn't the first time my life has been threatened. When I was 15, I was told I would probably die from cancer. Miraculously, through loads of chemo and radiation – I survived. It was scary then, but it's much scarier now.

I look at my four sons, one who is only just four months old, and I wonder if I will be able to survive cancer again. Could I be that lucky? Will I be there for my sons? To pick them up when they fall, to watch their successes and failures as they become men, graduate, get married, and have children? Will a new woman lie beside my boyfriend in a few years time; me just a dear memory hanging behind glass on a wall? I have so much more to lose now than when I was 15. I fear I've been living on borrowed time. Maybe it's come back to finish what it started so long ago. Will I ever be free from this constant dread of death hunting me? I'm so paralysed with fear. I don't want to die! I know I have to one day, but not now. Not even soon. I wish I could run away, take a drug, or get really, really drunk then wake up with a stinking headache the next day and realise it was all a bad dream.

If you believe in God, please pray for me. If you don't, please think of me and send positive energy my way. I need strength. I need to beat this demon – whatever it turns out to be. I hope that I will write again and tell you how silly I've been, but today all I can muster is this pitiful groping for a stick to hang onto before I'm swept away. It's a powerless place to be.

One week later, I am sitting in a modest office in the Nuffield Hospital again. Mr Zammit comes in, sits down slowly in front of me, remains silent for a moment and then begins. Speaking gently in a hushed tone he says, 'It is cancer I'm afraid,' laying his hand flat on his desk like a silent gavel coming down following a verdict. Sat closely next to me, Peter squeezes my knee.

Mr Zammit, Pam, and Peter wait silently for my reaction. There is none. I just blink and play my usual game of hide and seek with my emotions. Mr Zammit continues, 'We don't have all the information back from the pathologist yet, but I do have enough to be certain it is cancer. You will need treatment as soon as possible.' Treatment? That gets my attention.

'What kind of treatment?' I ventured – knowing damn well what that meant.

'First we'd like to start you on chemotherapy, followed by surgery and then radiotherapy.'

The word chemotherapy finally gets a quivering lip as I recall the chemotherapy I went through years ago, but I think they are all still stunned by how well I was handling the news.

'What kind of surgery?'

A very long pause ensues.

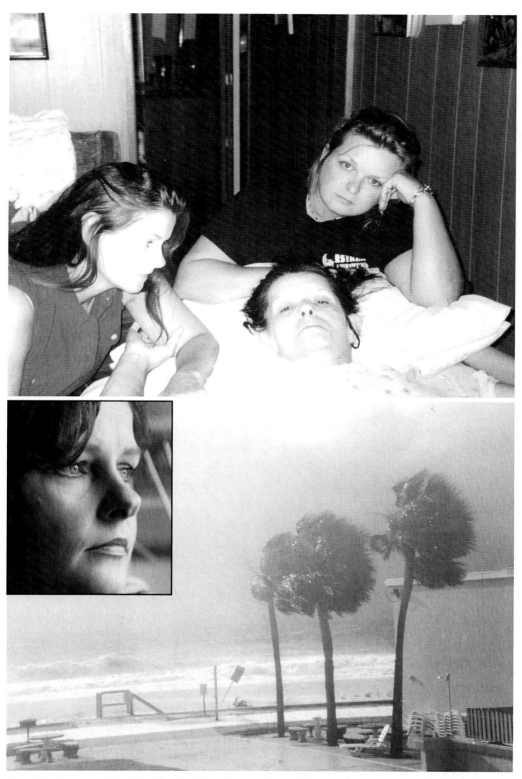

Top: Me, Terry and Sheila–The last time I would see Terry
Bottom: On leaving the hospital, a hurricane began to brew

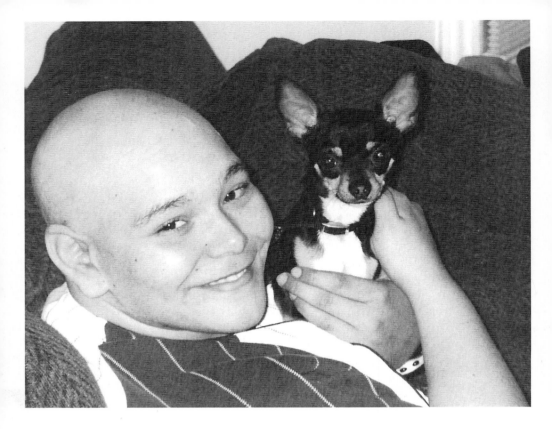

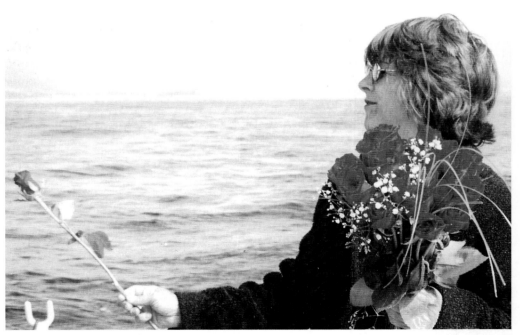

Top: Kay going through treatment
Bottom: Mom with roses after scattering Kay's ashes

'A mastectomy.'

The words ricochet off my face. Staring at him blankly and trying to heavily blink away threatening tears, my mind is still computing what that means, repeatedly spelling it out. Finally, the syllables string themselves together and reach my processing centre. I can't hold it any longer; sobbing, I fall into Peter's lap. I simply can't face the world – I need to hide my face, fear, and pain.

Pam immediately leaves the room to get me some water I didn't ask for and don't drink. Everybody waits silently, touching me on my leg or squeezing my hand, waiting for me to pull myself together so the conversation can continue – because it must. My sobs eventually die down to normal tears, and Mr Zammit continues to explain what will happen next. He has already arranged for me to see a colleague, an Oncologist, that evening. In the meantime, I need to go downstairs immediately and have scans and X-rays performed. He ends by saying he knows it will be difficult, but it is necessary to have all of the treatment because 'what you don't want to have to do is go through this again. Isn't it?' I soon learned Mr Zammit ends many of his sentences with 'isn't it?' even when it doesn't make sense. It's part of his charm.

Escorted out of Mr Zammit's office, Peter pushes my 4-month-old son ahead in his pushchair, while Mr Zammit follows behind rubbing my shoulder. As nice as the gesture is, I don't look back. I wish I could, but there is no looking back now.

We follow Pam downstairs to the imaging department where another nurse takes over. She asks me to please undress. As she begins explaining which way around to wear the robe she has given me, I begin to sob again.

'Do you want me to stop, or shall I just push on?'

'No, No… it's OK, please continue,' I say politely in a small voice, as if I really have a choice. I can no longer employ my usual trick of wait and see if the situation will sort itself. In this case, that isn't an option.

First I have an ultra sound and then a mammogram. The nurse places my diseased breast between two cold metal plates and squeezes them together very tightly. It hurts. It really, really hurts. When she releases my breast, there is some sort of ooze left behind. She says that it's normal and asks me to sit down and wait in the small room while they review the images to make sure all is OK, which clearly it isn't. I sit alone for what seems an eternity having just been told I have cancer. Again. Tears sting my eyes and streak my cheeks. I want Peter. I wish he were sat next to me now.

Next I am taken to the X-ray department where images are taken of my lungs. I haven't even considered my lungs or the rest of my body until now. Immediately thoughts of my little sister flood my mind; the times before she died when she coughed up pieces of her lungs and thought it was funny to show me. I wonder suddenly if I will go the same way, and if she felt anything like I did now. Did she feel an unforgiving and unrelenting loneliness in the fact that she may die? She probably didn't because she believed in God. I wonder how I could ever believe in God with the way my life has tortured me.

Fortunately the nurse is able to assure me that as far as she can tell my lungs are clear. In a matter of minutes it had dawned on me that it could be in my lungs to finding out it wasn't. My head and emotions are spinning. I feel sick and dizzy.

On our arrival home, Peter's mother who had been looking after our boys awaited our news. Up to this point, she had insisted that I didn't have cancer. I found it irritating because I felt she was making light of my fears. Therefore, one small part of me, the rebellious teenager, wanted to stick two fingers up and say, 'See! I told you it was cancer!' My victory is short lived as I hear only one person's applause in my mind slowly and unenthusiastically, *Clap... clap... clap... Well done, Lora Lee. You are the winner,* I say to myself. Except in this case, I didn't want to be.

Later that day, at 6 PM an Oncologist's secretary leads Peter and me into an office at the Nuffield Hospital. Dr Richard Simcock extends a hand and a warm, soft hello. *Oh wow – he's young,* I note to myself. I didn't expect that. I don't know what I expected — probably Dr Hardy. We shake hands and take our seats. Dr Simcock begins by saying I can call him Richard if I like, or Dr Simcock – whatever makes me happy. *What would make me happy is if I didn't have to call on you at all,* I scream at him in my mind.

'As Mr Zammit explained to you earlier today, you have breast cancer.'

This was the second time somebody said that to me, but it still felt like the first. My eyes began to water.

Dr Simcock went through great effort to carefully and cautiously explain what he knows about my tumours, 'What Mr Zammit wasn't able to tell you about your cancer, which I now can, is that your tumours are Grade 2, hormone receptive, 3.5 and 1.5 cm, Stage 3,' blah blah blah!

I stopped listening, and thought, *'There's that cancer word again. No, no, no cancer, think about his nice pen. Think about how old he is. Does he always work this late? I can see he's married – wonder if he has children. I wonder how my children are...'*

Next thing I hear is that for the next year, my life will be taken over by medical treatment.

Fading out again, I take stock: he's tall and thin with short blond hair, longish sideburns and down turned eyes. He is very calm and methodical as he explains things. I think, *I'm not mentally defective just because I have cancer you know!* I look at his tie – nice. I look at his office – big. I look at his Blackberry – impressive. I look at Peter's shoes – *he needs new shoes, I really must buy him some new shoes.* I look out through the hospital window and think of the nights when I was in my cell at Hillcrest Juvenile Hall where I would lay dreaming of my freedom. I shout at myself, *stop it Lora Lee! You aren't 15 anymore! You are a grown woman who has just been told you have cancer again. You really must pay attention; this is serious.*

Reluctantly, I force myself back to thoughts in the room and concentrate just in time to hear him say that he understands I am probably feeling a little bewildered and overwhelmed, so he is going to try to keep it short this evening. He pops a tape into a machine and pushes RECORD. Forty-five minutes later, he pushes STOP, takes the tape out, turns it over, and presses RECORD once again. Another forty-five minutes later the tape runs out, but my questions have not. I am now fully present and ready to take on board as much as I can.

It is now around 7:30 pm and Dr Simcock says I must be weary, so we will call it a night. I think he is weary of all my questions! He writes me out a prescription for the pain I am experiencing in my breast, there isn't one for the ache my heart, and I ask him one final question: 'What are my chances of survival?'

Dr Simcock hesitates. He pulls himself away from me while sucking in a deep breath, almost as if trying to decide if he should tell me. 'OK' he says letting his breath go in a huff. He grabs his Blackberry and takes me to 'Adjuvant Online,' a website designed to give doctors and their patients some idea of their likely outcome. He explains that based on one positive node in my axilla (armpit), if I just have surgery with no chemo, I have around 67% chance of survival. If I have both surgery and chemo, it jumps to 76%. If I have surgery, chemo, radiotherapy, and hormone treatment, my chances of survival are around 82%. As it happens, these figures are irrelevant to me because they are based on ductal breast cancer, not inflammatory breast cancer that I was diagnosed with. Subsequently my chances of survival are as low as 40%.

The following morning around 8:00 AM, the telephone rings. Blurry-eyed and exhausted from no sleep the night before, I answer the phone.

'Hello?'

'Hi Lora Lee, it's Richard.'

I think, *Who?*

'Richard Simcock' he says noticing my delay in reply.

'Oh, hi' said with a long 'i' to muster the slightest sound of enthusiasm.

'Just wondering how you are coping. Did you get any sleep last night?'

'No. I'm not feeling very well. I feel numb, and can't stop thinking.'

He says without a moment's hesitation, 'You're ruminating. Next time, if you don't fall asleep within 20 minutes, get up, write down whatever is worrying you, and then try to sleep again in half an hour. The more you try to focus on how you can't sleep, the less likely you will be able to.'

'Oh...OK...'

There's a long pause on the other end of the line.

'Lora Lee, It's going to take some time to come to terms with your diagnosis. May I suggest we meet up again so we can re-cap?'

'Sure. OK. When?'

Without realising it, I had just jumped aboard the never-ending appointment treadmill that would become my life for the next year and more. The next appointment was a bone scan in Hove, then an ECG to check my heart function — also in Hove, but on another day. Following this, I had a meeting with the Chemotherapy nurses at Brighton General Hospital in the Chemo Suite. Whilst I waited for a nurse, Dr Simcock rushed into the room, not the same calm man I met a week ago, but a rather hyper and rushed man. He said hello, and we had a small chat. Then he disappeared as quickly as he had arrived.

A couple of days later and I had another meeting with Dr Simcock to discuss the findings from the scans. Back at the Nuffield, he was once again calm and methodical. I found the variance in his behaviour difficult, it was hard enough coping with my own emotional vicissitudes let alone my doctor's. I soon learned that when he was at the NHS hospital, he was swept off his feet, rushing around trying to get it all done, but at the Nuffield, he had more time with his patients. I also quickly learned when I had asked a question that made him uncomfortable. He would immediately try to divert attention from his discomfort by picking up an imaginary object or piece of fluff off the floor – swooping down quickly so I was unable to register the expression on his face.

Following our meeting, I was feeling more positive because I had found out that my body was clear of cancer except for my left breast and lymph node in my armpit. I was very relieved to have all the tests and waiting over with so that I could concentrate on surviving breast cancer. Now that I knew the full scale of my demon, I could put my boxing gloves on and start the fight.

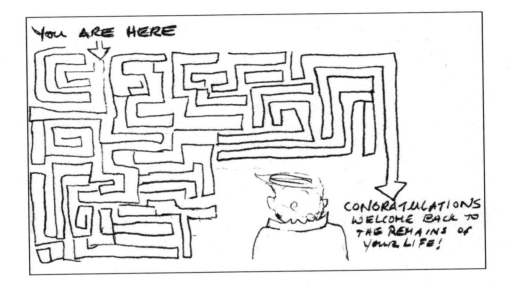

Chapter 38

Reaction

Being told for the second time I had an illness that could potentially end my life had a funny way of putting things into perspective, and suddenly my priorities seemed much clearer. I became achingly aware of things in my life that weren't quite right. Namely, I had a huge hole in my soul brought on by loneliness and I didn't know how to fill it or make it better. Facing this pain was a battle in itself, let alone surviving cancer. I began to think, *'If I'm going to die, is this how I want to go?'* I wondered if maybe this loneliness is what caused my cancers in the first place. I began to believe that I had to embrace my past if I was to move forward from the prison I was in and conquer cancer.

My driving forces were my four beautiful sons. I have so much more to do in their lives. I wasn't going to allow breast cancer to get in the way. Instead, I promised myself I was going to see breast cancer as my wake up call to get the most from my life and to correct the things that I'd been letting slide for too long. I didn't want to sweat the small stuff anymore – it had already wasted too much time and detracted from what was important. Of course very much part of that was my relationship with my children's father. This is my family, and I would do anything to make sure we stayed together.

Another minor factor that motivated me was that I didn't want to feel like a parcel anymore. I had spent my entire life having my destiny dictated to me by outside forces, so I was determined to take control and steer my life the way I wanted and needed it to go. I couldn't allow cancer to take and remain in control of my life.

As I have done so many times in my life when things were too difficult to bear, I started writing in a journal to express some of the fears and emotional issues that cancer had brought up. On my opening page I wrote:

> *'I see my story ending with Peter and I watching our sons grow up, graduate, get married and settle into careers. Be it my will alone, they will have a great deal of happiness and love in their lives. I will be there when they start school, learn to ride a bike, go on their first date. I will be there whether they are laughing or crying. God help me, I will be there whenever they need me to lean on, to provide safety and security in a harsh and cruel world. They need mommy cuddles and tickles and to know that they are fabulous no matter what they do, say or wear. I need Peter and them too... we are all very much in this together.'*

The lead up to being told I had breast cancer, and indeed the proceeding couple of weeks, I felt so powerless and out of control. I had cancer, and there wasn't much I could do but go with the flow. Except there were some things I could do psychologically to make my preparation for the treatment ahead a bit more bearable. The first thing I did after purchasing my journal (and subsequently a beautiful pen from Mont Blanc that became my best friend), was spend a fortune on skincare products designed to protect my skin from the damaging effects of free radicals caused by chemo and radiotherapy. This made me feel better emotionally, and I hoped they really were protecting my skin. I also bought two wigs for the day my hair began to fall out, and some new clothes that would help me feel better in the difficult days to come.

I also bought an arsenal of books believing knowledge is power. Cancer once was hard enough. Cancer twice was enough – no more – this was it! I was going to run Cancer's butt out of town for the very last time, and he wouldn't be coming back in any shape or form. I bought nearly every single cancer book there is and dutifully read them one by one. The end result is that it nurtured my fighting spirit and gave me back the feeling of being a little more in control.

Chapter 39

Treatment

In the early days of treatment, I had this overwhelming urge to throw myself at Dr Simcock in floods of tears and beg him to understand and make me better. Like a frightened and vulnerable little girl, I wanted a parent to hold me, to be able to bury my head into strong arms against a broad chest and feel protected. He fit that role. He was in a position to be strong and detached so that I could be weak for a moment, and I didn't even have to deal with any of his garbage as a person. I would attend my appointment, he would give me his undivided attention, and I would walk away feeling like the only patient he had. He was my knight in shining armour, and I was a damsel in distress.

I wouldn't say Dr Simcock is unattractive; he just isn't the Robert Redford come Sir Lancelot that I made him into in my mind. The doctor that originally appeared to me an average person suddenly became the most handsome and wonderful man in the whole world. I would have done anything to please him, to ensure he would look after and save me.

At one point, I dragged my entire family along to a meeting with Dr Simcock – half out of necessity (no babysitter) and half out of blackmail. I wanted him to see first hand what was at stake so that maybe he'd dig that much deeper into his knowledge and make it all better. The rational side of me knew this was an unfair pressure to put on any person – after all, he is just human. Then the emotional, desperate side of me wanted to control the situation. I wished enough charm and questions would ensure a positive outcome. Unfortunately he couldn't guarantee me this, nor can any doctor his patient diagnosed with such an illness, and this was a very hard pill to swallow. I did feel confident, however, that between his medical knowledge and my sheer will to survive, we would make a very good team. I just hoped I was a better patient for this doctor than I was for my last.

I had read somewhere that an American survey had proven difficult patients have better survival rates. When I told Dr Simcock about what I had read, he replied, 'Not difficult... challenging.' So although I didn't throw temper tantrums anymore, it would appear I still wasn't the ideal patient.

Dr Simcock explained my medical regime to me, that first I would have four cycles of 'FEC' (an acronym for Five Fluorouracil, Epirubicin, and Cyclophosphamide), followed by four cycles of Docetaxel all administered every 21 days. Following chemotherapy I would have surgery where they would remove my breast (a mastectomy), then a month or so after I would begin radiotherapy every day for five weeks, as well as start taking Tamoxifen. Tamoxifen is a drug that stops cancer cells from being able to dwell by jamming up the lock on the hormone receptors making it impossible for the cancer cells to open the lock, get in and feed. The theory being that with no hormones to feed on, the cancer cells would not be able to thrive.

It was explained that I would lose my hair, but I could try the Cold Cap in order to keep it for as long as possible. Nausea induced by chemotherapy would be minimised by use of steroids. Once treatment was finished, I had the choice of having Zoladex injections, which would stop my body from producing hormones by halting the production of eggs from my ovaries. Although all of this was a lot of information to take in, it seemed straightforward enough.

What wasn't immediately clear to me was the writing between the lines. I sat in my garden shortly after being diagnosed feeling shocked and dazed thumbing through pamphlets and books slowly realising that my world was going to change forever. Even once the cancer treatment had finished, I would never be the same. I read about how the chemotherapy drugs would most likely make me infertile once treatment started, sending me into an early menopause. The drugs may also cause me to develop Myeloid Leukaemia, and I could suffer a heart attack as a result of the Epirubicin. My bones may develop osteoporosis and there's a threat of cancer developing in my womb as a result of taking Tamoxifen. Not to mention I would lose my breast and have unsightly scars.

What I found most upsetting, however, was that breast cancer can return at any point no matter how long you've been in remission or cured. Therefore, although I may be ten years down the line cancer free, I will always be looking over my shoulder wondering if that pain or bump is indicative of something more sinister.

I had to make a decision. I asked myself if the misery I was about to endure would be worth it, and I easily reached an answer. Yes. Yes because this is life and I had to fight for it. Yes because I have a family that needs me. Yes because who knows what tomorrow may bring for any one of us. I wanted to be here to find out. There will only ever be one me, and I happen to like being me. I wasn't going to give away my life without a fight.

Physically I responded to the first couple of chemotherapy

treatments like a trooper. My doctor, Peter and Mom all kept warning me to take special care of myself because the chemotherapy drugs weakened my immune system. Unfortunately, this advice was lost on me and eventually I did pick up a cold from my children that normally I would have shrugged off. However, normal no longer, I struggled for a few nights to breathe despite having taken a flu and Actifed tablet. Luckily, it did stay as just a cold and didn't escalate into anything more serious. Considering that was the only illness during all of my treatment, I feel I was lucky compared to some.

The chemotherapy drugs had a short life span once mixed, therefore before my chemotherapy drugs were ordered at the hospital, I'd be given a blood test to check that my blood counts were all in the normal range. They always were, and considering how awful I felt emotionally, that always surprised me. Dr Simcock said that many patients mistakenly believe that if they feel bad emotionally their bodies are physically depressed too, which simply isn't the case. A patient can feel suicidal and their blood counts would be normal — believe me, I know.

The only difficulty the nurses encountered were my veins' lack of cooperation. As soon as I smelled rubbing alcohol, they once again disappeared altogether. This was no dress rehearsal; my veins knew what to do. As a result, after the second treatment, between the blood tests and the intravenous drips, my hands and arms were covered in purple splotches making me look like a drug addict. Dr Simcock recommended I have a Portacath inserted in the upper right side of my chest just below my collarbone that would lay under the surface of my skin and would connect to the jugular vein in my neck. The portacath would act as a permanent porthole to put needles into and deliver medicine or take bloods. I liked the idea that I didn't have to feel the cold medicine coursing up my arm anymore, and the drugs couldn't leave sore veins or track marks as they had previously.

The night before treatment they gave me steroids to help with the induced nausea the following day. The problem with steroids is that they kept me awake the night before treatment, the day of the treatment and for two days and nights following. When they finally started wearing off, the coming down stage would have me in floods of exhausted tears. I was too tired even to realise I was tired and would sit at the dining room table drinking wine, listening to music and crying inconsolably until 4 AM when I would finally fall asleep with my head on the table.

> **Blog:** *...Before I take steroids I now know to make a long list of things to do. Instead of sitting up all night listening to Patsy Cline, I could have had a steroidal clean house. Steroids are pure rocket fuel! Managing the extra horsepower coursing through my veins is like trying to walk a hungry tiger on a lead. Agitation and sleeplessness overwhelm coping capabilities. I like author Stephen White's description when he likened being on steroids to taking on characteristics of the Seven Dwarfs on amphetamines: 'Grumpy on Speed would be the dominant Dwarf. He – or in this case, she – would be around virtually the whole time, only reluctantly sharing the stage with Sleepy on Speed and Dopey on Speed. Sadly, Happy on Speed would make only the briefest of cameo appearances – usually taking place during a narrow window in the first act.' God I will miss steroids...*

On the day of treatment, I would have the Cold Cap tightly fitted to freeze my brain to a mind numbing -5 degrees Celsius. The theory being that if you stop the blood flow to the cells in your scalp, the chemotherapy drugs will not be able to reach them and be able to cause the damage which would cause hair to fall out.

Once I got over the treatment, chemo nausea and steroidal effects I went into denial mode. I couldn't quite distinguish if I was feeling 'positive' or if I was simply trying to forget. How could I ever forget though? Almost every other thought was *'God, will I be here in a year to see this again?'* – or – on more depressing days, it was *'I know I'm going to die. Who will look after my boys and love them the way I do?'* Then again, I had bad days where all the boys had colds, and I was feeling particularly under the weather with lack of sleep and I couldn't wait for them to go to bed. At times like that, I wondered if maybe somebody else would be a better mother than me.

Chapter 40

Functioning

Medically speaking, all was going as expected, but my emotional response and how I was functioning was a completely different matter altogether. My son Laurence was only four and a half months old when I started treatment, which meant long sleepless nights between waking up to feed him and me ruminating. I would wake in the night, and despite writing down my thoughts, I couldn't stop thinking. I wondered why I never thought that much when I had cancer so many years ago.

Exhausted most days, I found it difficult to function around the house but I had no choice but to continue to push myself. I had four boys who needed lunches made for nursery and school, dropping off and picking up, clean clothes to wear, bathing, feeding, stimulation and entertainment. Even though I needed rest, life demanded more and I wanted to be super Mom. As a result, my need to be alone increased, as did my moodiness. Ultimately my depression worsened.

When I did have help from Mom or Peter's mother, I was recovering from treatment so I never felt truly rested. As soon as I was physically able, I took the leads again. However, I wasn't the only one who was tired. Peter was being awakened in the night too and was exhausted by picking up the pieces. Mom would arrive from the States and the following day I'd have treatment all day so she wasn't even able to recover from her jet lag before taking care of the children from dawn to dusk. Then she wouldn't see me for days whilst I recovered from treatment. Not once did she, Peter or his mother complain. I know they must have felt the pressure as much as I did, but they bit their tongues and soldiered on.

> **Journal Entry:** *It's now two months into treatment and I am really struggling. I've taken a real nose-dive and am on a crying stint. I just get so frightened and feel so vulnerable. The smallest thing sets me off, and then I find it hard to snap back again. For me, the emotional roller coaster ride is far worse than the treatment itself. I'm finding it so very difficult to remain positive. I keep feeling like this is the end. What's upsetting me most right now is all the change; the fact that I have no control over matters and that I feel like just another statistic. I feel so un-special. I keep thinking of 'meat' for some reason. Everybody keeps telling me to call up a nurse and tell her all my feelings, but I just don't feel comfortable talking to strangers about my insecurities. It's the only thing private I have left anymore, and I don't want to lose that too.*
>
> *I have this overwhelming need and desire to be alone right now. Maybe it's depression, but I just want and need some peace and quiet. I want to think and sleep for a while, but there's <u>never</u> any let up with four boys and a partner. God, what will they do if anything happens to me? They can't or won't even let up a little for me now. Some mornings I don't even want to go downstairs because I know as soon as I do, everything is handed to me. I immediately have to handle the screaming children,*

empty the dishwasher, tidy the house, do the laundry... I just wish I could be ill for a while and somebody else could pick up the slack. Peter's mum is coming on Tuesday to help. Oh, I so wish I could go on holiday somewhere warm and just sleep, read, swim, bake and eat nice food. I'm tired of working so hard.

According to Dr Leslie Walker who has worked for more than 20 years on the mind-body approaches and improved survival in women with breast cancer, it's estimated that up to 77% of people with cancer are measurably depressed, which was a relief to learn, as I suddenly didn't feel so alone. Up to 45% of people who have undergone adjuvant chemotherapy (a mix of drugs like I had) are clinically diagnosed with some form of psychological or psychiatric disorder following treatment.

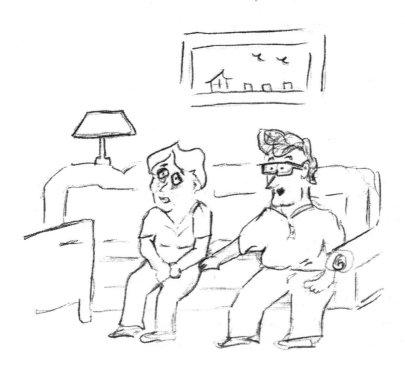

When I asked Dr Simcock if he felt 'emotional toxicity' (i.e., severe depression) can lead to cancer, his answer, like the loyal soldier ant bound to protect and serve his establishment, was that he's a scientist. He likes things he can measure. He said, 'You wouldn't be surprised to know that depressive symptoms are very common in patients with breast cancer but it doesn't mean that depression is a cause.'

Now, if I had asked him, 'Does depression suppress your oxygen levels, does this in turn have an impact on your immune system, and can that lead to cell misfunction?' his answer may have been different.

The effects of my cancer and subsequent treatment didn't end with me. As anticipated, PJ took the news hard and within two weeks of being back at school had two detentions for poor behaviour and his grades dropped. What I found most upsetting, however, is that he didn't want to come home at the weekends, preferring to stay at school or go to his dad's. He said it was because he had a cold and didn't want to infect me, but I suspect it was simply too much for him to see me so weak and vulnerable.

Tink was incredibly sweet, showing constant signs of worry for me. Unexpectedly he'd kiss me and ask me if I felt better. I think one of the most precious things he said was after I had my hair cut short in preparation of it falling out. He had said nothing of it the whole day. I thought he hadn't even noticed. Then, whilst kissing me goodnight, he said very sweetly, 'I love your hair, Mommy.' He was only three years old. I was so touched, I cried.

Jiggy was a bit confused about Peter's mother coming for three weeks immediately following a two week visit from our old Au Pair, then Mom coming straight after and staying for four weeks. His schedule was disturbed, but I hoped he was young and wouldn't remember. Indeed, that's what I told myself a lot when

I worried about the effect my cancer would have on them.

Laurence did the best out of all of my children because like a failing body that shuts down systematically to protect its vital organs to help it survive, I too focussed on the most needy putting him even before myself. He was the most vulnerable physically so he got more of my time.

Last but by no means least, there was of course Peter who felt an incredible pressure to provide and be strong for our family and me. He was so good at hiding his feelings I began to wonder if he had any at all. He retreated inside himself, and I felt that he was unhappy. At times, I felt a distinct annoyance with me for dragging our family down. I was now a constant burden for him while he tried to provide for the family I so desperately wanted and could possibly now abandon due to my illness. Sometimes I questioned if he was only staying with me out of a sense of duty. We had only been together seven years, known each other for nine, and so much had happened in such a short time. The stress must have been incredible for him; it certainly was for me. Although we had been through difficult times, never once did we imagine we'd be going through cancer together; at least, not this young. We had shared so many laughs, tender moments – even the odd explosive moment – but it was always OK. Suddenly it was no longer OK, and my relationship didn't feel safe.

Journal Entry: *I had a low point as I stood in the kitchen looking out into our garden. I watched Peter mowing the lawn with Tink two steps behind pushing his toy mower mimicking everything his daddy did. It was a sight that I have seen many times before, but today it caught me off guard and all I could do was think of how much I love Peter and how I've waited so long to have him in my life. I really don't want it taken away now. He deserves so much more. I do so hope that I'm*

the one there for the rest of his life. I can't help but cry.
I feel so powerless. I've never known I could love like this.
It makes me happy and saddens me all at once. I feel
frightened for us. We are so good together. I just get so
sad when I think of the worse case scenario. When I start
crying and worrying like this, I feel like a traitor. I'm
supposed to remain positive and take it on the chin. God
only knows if love was enough to pull me through this,
there'd be no problem.

I worried a lot about Peter throughout my treatment. I worried what he would think of me when I lost my hair, or that he might wish he'd never bet on this horse. I worried that he was going to have a breakdown with all the stress. I needed his constant reassurance that everything was going to be all right, but no doubt this just added to his pressures.

One night I was feeling particularly needy of his attention and simply couldn't settle down. 'Honey, look at me' I said. When he did I snapped his photo. He looked at me with dead annoyance. I took another snap and he held up his magazine in front of his face and told me to go away.

'Can I have a back rub?' I asked plonking myself on the couch next to him – demanding he touch me. He let out a long sigh, and proceeded to rub my shoulders while he watched the television. After a short while he stopped, and still seeking affection I jumped up, left the room and returned with my two wigs.

'What do you think of this one honey?' I asked modelling the short blonder one.

'Yes, it looks good on you,' he said looking at me very briefly and returning his gaze to the television.

I knew I had to do something else because this tactic wasn't working. I took my brown shoulder length wig and put it on his head. He sat patiently like an old dog being roughed up by a toddler. 'Oh look! It's just like when you were a teenager in the 70's!' I said while he sat and blinked at me impatiently.

'Look, I just want some time to myself OK?' he said with irritation as I continued to do cartwheels to get his attention.

This was the beginning of a rocky road ahead. One where we were both trying to be strong for each other and ourselves but at the same time completely alienating one another from the support we should been sharing as a couple.

It wasn't just Peter retreating into himself. I knew Peter was feeling the strain, often saying 'What about me?' I was completely self -absorbed trying to keep my act together, pushing him aside and not giving him the warmth he needed. I didn't know how to explain that although I love him, I needed to take care of myself. I was scrambling to find my way and at the same time trying to nurture my fighting spirit. The energy and guidance I needed was from myself and other people, other than my family and him entirely. In order to be there for my boys and him in the future, I needed to go alone through the painful process I was in. I wanted to be fit and strong for them again one day, so I tore myself down so I could rebuild a stronger me. I was allowing all my pent up emotions to come flooding back and was exposing a raw, vulnerable side to me that I wasn't used to sharing so I pushed him away.

Ultimately I was frightened of hurting Peter either by dying, or with the thoughts and feelings I was experiencing. I had no control over my emotions and I felt intensely guilty that my mind wasn't always thinking the things it should. Not getting enough attention and affection at home, Sir Lancelot began playing a bigger role in my imagination, and I was letting Peter and my family down. Sometimes I cared, and sometimes I didn't. There was such a huge part of me that just wanted some freedom and space to do and be something other than a woman going through breast cancer, or a mother going through breast cancer, or a wife going though breast cancer. I wanted to dance, sing, travel, create beautiful art and write amazingly inspiring words, but all that kept coming out was pain. My sorrow was so intense; I kept saying I was going to make it through this, but my heart believed something else, and no matter how hard I tried, I couldn't hide from my fear and feelings. It was driving me insane. I wanted to run away, but one foot in front of the other was all I could manage – let alone running or dancing!

I wondered when it would all happen for me, when would I feel happy and content? At what point would I believe I was OK and stop worrying? How would I know when I'd reached the point where I could relax again? Who would I be at the end of this journey? Who would I touch and who would I hurt? When would my thoughts and feelings ever be good enough? I was frightened of who I was and who I might become. I felt everything I ever knew about myself was eroding away. I was tired and lonely. I wished I could feel love, love for Peter, but all I felt was panic and stress. I had to believe it would change. Otherwise, what was the point in going on? There was so much going on in my mind, and I feared for my relationship that my heart wouldn't find its way.

Poem written to Peter

Different Seasons

Laughter! Heart pounding, worldliness, wild tempo!
A celebration and toast to life
Beautiful, strong, pure, together
Unstoppable, untouchable – the envy of most

Heads once held high proudly singing
Fall lower and steady
Weight gaining in grey clouds lingering
Salty luke-warm drops unearth buried truths

I feel fear and passion like thunderous footsteps
Enter my open mind
Trampling my idea of love before
Nothing but pulsing hurt and wanting ego once more

Who am I now?
Drenched in weight and sorrow
Take deep breaths, sop yourself up, walk on and be proud!
You are courage, hope and inspiration to some

However shadows and darkness may threaten
A new day dawns giving rise to sunny beginnings.
I hear whispering promises of love and fairy tales
I am here my darling, however reduced, nothing less, wishing for more

You are not forgotten; you are a beautiful song
A smile on tender lips, giving voice to untold spring
Hearts frozen in the moment begin to melt
Intense love, joy and laughter continue to echo even if I sleep.

Chapter 41

Anger

Once I was over the initial shock and had accepted my treatment regime, I became angry towards everything and everybody. I was angry that my body was letting me down, especially when I felt so strong. I was tired of people who promised the world to me trying to be supportive and helpful, but not really being there when I needed them most. I was angry with myself that I wasn't more interested in having cancer. All I could think was, *this sucks!* That's deep. Nevertheless, it did suck (excuse my American slang), and my true feelings, as always, were protected by lots of denial and anger.

I was angry too with Sheila who talked to me once on the phone after my diagnosis and then nothing, not even emails, during all of my treatment. I knew from my first experience of having cancer that everybody's reaction to learning a loved one has cancer is different, but I couldn't understand how my own sister could once again cut me off completely during such a difficult time in my life. She was acting exactly like Terry, running when things got too tough, and that made me even angrier.

I also felt angry that my home was being taken over by visitors and that I was suddenly being left outside decisions on how to run my home because nobody wanted to stress me. I wondered if that was really the reason, or was it more convenient and easier to do what they wanted if I was out of the way? I'd come downstairs from my bedroom and go to do something only to be told, 'That's not how we do it now. We do it like this...' Even more irritating, 'He doesn't like that food now – he likes this...'

One night following treatment, I came downstairs to join Peter and his mother for dinner. They were so engrossed in their discussion, they didn't even acknowledge my presence. I registered it but said nothing. They continued talking while we all sat down for a meal prepared by his mother. I sat in my usual spot at the head of the table and they sat next to each other.

'Excuse me, can you pass the salt please?' I interjected in between a short pause in their conversation. There was no reply, no salt was handed to me, and their conversation continued. I reached for the salt myself.

'What are you guys talking about?'

Once again there was no reply. 'Excuse me!' I said loudly getting their attention. They both looked at me like I had a spade sticking out of my head.

'I was just wondering' I didn't even finish the sentence before his mother cut me off again. 'Oh for God's sake! Nobody is fucking listening to me!' I shouted and threw my napkin on the table before storming back up to bed.

I was also angry that every time I turned around I was advised on what to eat and even what to wear. It made me bitter that it was constantly implied that I'd done something to deserve having breast cancer. If it wasn't my poor 'Western Diet,' it was what I put on my skin, what I drank, my poor mental state of mind, and my genes. Somehow, it was always my fault, and if I wanted to survive, I should eat a strict diet; otherwise, I'm 'out of here' (dead) – no cheating allowed! All of a sudden, life really stank and was wholly trying. And 'don't eat that piece of toast with butter or you'll die!' Well, honestly… if life was going to be so dull and unhappy all the time – who wanted to live anyways? I'm not saying a healthy diet isn't a good idea, just that there should be balance and moderation. All work and no play makes any person go insane.

Another thing that irritated me even more than a screaming two year old was when I heard or read about women who claimed they'd never asked, 'Why me?' when they found out they had breast cancer. Well, I guess that makes many other women, including me, look like real complainers, doesn't it?

Everybody kept telling me I'd be fine, and until I was diagnosed with breast cancer myself, I always thought very little of it — especially as it is so 'common and treatable.' I always assumed whoever had breast cancer would be fine. That's how it was until I was told I had it, then suddenly it became a lot more real and frightening, and I found myself getting angry at people that, just as I did, assumed I'd be alright.

One evening whilst Mom was visiting, I had too much wine and all my anger erupted in a spew of toxic venom. Mom had said that she couldn't understand why I always felt unloved by her – that she loves me very much. If she didn't, why would she have given up so much time to come and help my family and me during such a difficult time? Misdirecting all my pent up rage at having cancer again, I struck out at her like a rattlesnake hissing, 'Well, maybe it has something to do with falling asleep at Grandmas listening to you shout, *I hate her Bob, I hate her!*'

It was a mean and low dig, but I didn't care because I was hurting inside and I wanted the whole world to know. The next day she asked me to please forgive her for saying that – she couldn't even recall the circumstances. I felt ashamed I had brought it up. It was so long ago and irrelevant to our relationship now. Looking back, I believe I chose her to vent my anger on because finally at age 37, I knew she wouldn't abandon me.

Another thing that made me want to kick and punch the air in extreme annoyance was when well meaning people kept telling me how strong and brave I am. Like I had a choice. I asked myself repeatedly what made me so 'courageous?' When Dr Simcock told me I was dealing with treatment so well in his eyes – what does that mean when I was obviously coming apart at the seams? I was a certifiable wacko who needed a straight jacket, and yet he told me how well I was handling the situation and how strong I am!

Then one day I had an episode with Tink at Eastbourne Emergency Paediatric Department that made it clearer in my mind why I was, indeed, so brave. Unfortunately, Tink had a very high temperature and tummy pains, and the last two attempts to sort him out through our General Practitioner had failed, so I brought him to the hospital. They decided to take a blood test, which he'd never had before. Once it was all over, and believe me it was very traumatic, I said 'Well done, son. What a brave boy!'

'No I'm NOT! I was frightened!' he said through thick tears.

I thought about it for a moment and replied, 'Yes, even though you were frightened you still allowed them to do it and that's what makes you so very brave.' It dawned on me I had answered one of my own mysteries. What makes me so brave? Now I know, I am brave because even though I was frightened of treatment, even though I knew it would hurt me emotionally and physically,

I allowed them to do what they needed to do in order to survive. When I told Dad my revelation, he said, 'and by saying what you did, you gave him permission to cry – that it's OK. I want you to know that even though you are brave, you are also allowed to cry sometimes too.'

'*Courage is being scared to death, but saddling up anyway.*'
John Wayne, Actor

Chapter 42

Disappointed and frightened

After my third cycle of FEC, I had a second ultrasound scan to see if my tumours had reduced or changed. When I got the news for the second time that there was no noted change, my heart felt heavy, like my demon of an opponent was winning.

I walked upstairs in the Nuffield Hospital, holding back my grief as I headed into Dr Simcock's office to discuss the findings. Dr Simcock bounded in behind me and I felt my heart sink even further. Not only was I letting myself and my family down but also my dedicated, caring doctor. I sat down in the chair to the side of his desk, and he sat down on his wheelie chair behind it asking me how the scan went as he did. I answered by crying, explaining that I was just tired. I didn't tell him I was tired of living – tired of all the ups and downs; tired of feeling positive one moment then having hope pulled out from under me the next. In a heartbeat he had pushed himself out from behind his desk stopping just in front of me. He held his arms out open wide – legs spread apart in an unconscious 'come to daddy' gesture.

Quickly his body language changed. He crossed his legs and arms and leaned back in his chair, obviously distancing himself emotionally from the situation at hand. He patiently explained that this is the reason they wanted to try chemotherapy before surgery; they (meaning Mr Zammit and Dr Simcock) wanted to make sure the drugs actually had an effect on my cancer before they removed the tumours. Now that they knew FEC was having minimal effect, they were going to change to Docetaxel, cutting the number of treatments I was to receive down by one.

During our meeting, Mr Zammit came in. They both wanted a look at my breast. I said, 'It's OK, I'm getting used to taking my top off now.' Dr Simcock looked down and shuffled some stuff around on his desk with an embarrassed smile. I didn't mean to imply he was a pervert. I was just feeling mouthy and down.

Then I went to the hospital bed and Pam pulled the curtain around so I could have some amount of privacy before I took off my top. When I said I was ready, both Mr Zammit and Dr Simcock came behind the curtain joining Pam and me. Assuming the usual position, I laid down and Mr Zammit took charge by telling me to please sit up.

Both men stood back against the curtain, staring at my breasts as if they were looking at wheels on a car — first one, then the other. Mr Zammit asked me to raise my arms above my head as they talked about the appearance of my breasts as if I wasn't there or attached to them. It went something along the lines of, 'Look Richard,' as Mr Zammit pointed, 'the skin on the affected breast looks much better. Do you remember it looked like an orange peel before with large pores?'

'I didn't see her when it looked like that. By the time I saw her, the inflammation had gone down, but you're right, it does look like there's been some improvement.' Dr Simcock said with crossed arms and hand held to his chin in a thinking gesture. Meanwhile, I sat there trying not to die from embarrassment.

I was asked to lie down and the hard probing of Mr Zammit began. He kept referring to Dr Simcock, and Dr Simcock kept rubbing his hands together probably in an effort to warm them, but it looked strangely like a child who couldn't wait to get his hands in the cookie jar. Dr Simcock repeatedly asked if he could have a feel. Finally Mr Zammit allowed Dr Simcock his turn, and more probing continued. He said he was pleased with how the tumour felt. Apparently it had softened quite a bit and they both agreed they were happy with 'it'. 'The change hasn't been brilliant but is very promising,' they both tried to reassure me, but it didn't work.

Following the meeting, I sat at home on my bed facing my truths. I wasn't particularly proud of how I'd been coping. I was drinking myself stupid instead of writing or talking about my feelings. It was just so boring and hard to live and breathe cancer all the time. I was using alcohol to forget, like Terry did throughout her life. I felt like I could drink my way through the entire experience, but knew it wasn't the answer. My poor body was going through enough without poisoning it every night. I really needed to get my act together.

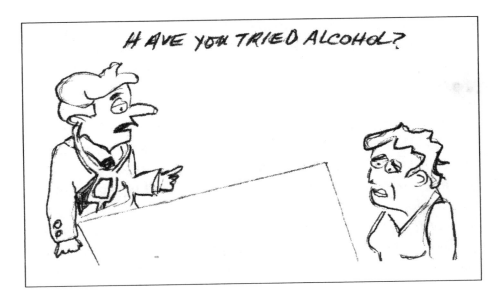

BLOG – 'Much Ado About Nothing!': *What a load of hooo – haaa for nothing! Just found out last night that the three rounds of chemo I've received have barely touched my tumours. I can't believe that all this chemo taking, green tea drinking, supplement taking, blueberry eating, positive thinking, no dairy, organic diet mumbo jumbo has made no difference what so ever! Yeah, I'm feeling a little scared. And when I'm not feeling scared, I'm feeling panicky... and when it's not panicking on the menu, it's anger being served up in great big dollops... and when I'm asleep and wake in the middle of night, it's sheer loneliness when the same thought pops into my head that I may die. I can't remember the last time I felt happy. I'm always struggling with the before mentioned.*

I went alone to my scan last night. Probably the first time I've actually been physically alone since I found out I have breast cancer. After the news of 'no noted change', I drove home in the dark and allowed myself to cry deeply. Do you know what it's like to be told you may die, to imagine the world going on without you, your children growing up not knowing you? I only get one chance at this, and it seems nothing I do is making it any better. I feel so powerless. I'm not used to being out of control.

I came home and cried in Peter's arms and said through thick tears and great insistence, 'Tell them to help me! Tell them to make me better!' Why is this happening to me... again? I'm a good person. What am I supposed to be doing differently than I do now? And, of course, I continually ask God why He is doing this to me. I'm so tired. My life is too hard, and I wonder where I'll get the energy to beat this... I think it's fair to say; I'm having a terrible, rotten, no good, very bad day!

Although the tumours in my breast and lymphatic system were stable (not growing), they hadn't shrunk. Feeling very discouraged, I went into a self-pity funk. I wrote in my journal:

> *'To be quite honest, there are times when I think of the long path ahead of me, and the lifelong implications, and I start feeling maybe I'd rather not go on. That's hard to admit, and I'm not sure how long the thought hangs around before being replaced by dread and fear of not being there for my boys in the future. If it weren't for them, my willpower and drive to recover wouldn't be so strong. Frankly, I am tired. My life has been one struggle and survival after another. Nobody ever said life would be easy – nobody said it would be this difficult either.*

> *I suppose we all plod along looking for a special meaning to make it all worthwhile and not in vane. My reason is my family. I would be nothing without them. And so I keep trying, keep praying, keep eating stuff I can't stand in the name of survival, in the name of life, and hope that will give me more time with my boys big and small. Not for my sake, but theirs. I would never dream of not being there for them when they need me, as I know they'd always be there for me if they could. It makes me sad that with my past it has taken me so long to understand the true joy of family – only to have it threatened. I am desperate not to leave my children motherless like Terry did, but I'm so tired.*

> *Is this depression speaking? Fucking sucks all of this. I don't feel like playing anymore. There's nothing to look forward to. Except what? Maybe more cancer because of all the radiation and chemo they gave me this and last time?*

*Alternatively, how about a massive heart attack instead – also as a result of the Adriamycin I've received. Or, how about acute Leukaemia (yes, same reasons)? What are all benefits of this again? When will it all be worth it? Who gives a shit anyways? Yeah, having a **BAD** day.'*

Dr Rosy Daniel writes,

Looking at your will to live: The nitty gritty issue for anyone facing a life-threatening diagnosis is the question of how strong is your will to live? This is a highly confrontational question, but a vital one to nail if you are going to succeed in fighting cancer. Carl Jung realised many years ago that all of us have an equal and opposite urge towards life (eros) and towards death (thanetos). When the eros side is strong, we feel powerful and passionate towards life. But when thanetos is dominant, death can seem very seductive.

I woke up the following morning remembering a few things that made me feel much better. The first being that as a result of treatment, I was also going through menopause (one of the side effects of chemotherapy), so all of my feelings were exemplified 10 fold. Secondly, I had a large, hard tumour in my breast. It was unrealistic of me to expect dramatic changes with such a thriving mass. My tumour had softened and hadn't grown; I remembered that was the most important thing. Thirdly, I realised having sent a very urgent and upsetting 'SOS Blog' on Myspace, that through my hard core honesty and selfishness in the moment, I managed to upset many family members and friends who were travelling this journey with me. I decided I would be more careful in the future about just how much I shared, because although I woke up feeling much better – there were many more who were still picking themselves up and trying to recover from the hard truths I so easily blurted out.

I oscillated frequently in between understanding the process I was in, and struggling to make sense of anything at all. The more I tried to do and be, the less I accomplished and became. My body trembled with physical and emotional weariness until I nearly had an emotional breakdown. I simply couldn't function in the most basic of ways. Because I had grown very attached to Dr Simcock, Sir Lancelot of my fantasy world, who always seemed to have the right answers and who had filled a nurturing and caring role in my life, I emailed his secretary secretly hoping that he would come to my rescue and make it all better:

> *Hi Barbara, I am emailing you because I know how busy Dr Simcock is and I don't want to bother him.* (Yes I did. That's exactly what I wanted. I wanted him to drop everything and rush to my side.) *I've been in a bit of a funk the last few days. I feel really depressed and anxious. I keep having heart palpitations; I feel like I'm about to have a heart attack. I don't feel right and just wanted to be in contact with somebody to reassure me. I feel exhausted and don't feel like doing anything or being around anybody. There's no let up at home and I wish everybody would just leave me alone for a while! I generally feel like I can't do this. I wish I could check myself into a hotel room for a week and rest. The most worrying thing is how I feel like any moment I'm going to completely lose it! Any suggestions? Physically my body is low, and I'd be very surprised if my bloods are good enough for chemo on Thurs., but we'll just have to see. I am worried about myself. I don't like talking to people I don't know, and I really doubt talking is going to help me right now. I am a trained counsellor myself, so you'd think I could get my own head straight, eh? Right, sorry to lay that on you but any help you can suggest will be greatly appreciated. Kind regards, Lora Lee*

I didn't hear from Dr Simcock at this point, but received an unexpected call from my GP to check how I was coping. I don't know to this day if Dr Simcock had something to do with that, I'm sure he most likely did, but it came just in time. She told me I was no good in that state and to double my anti-depressants, which I did immediately. By the end of the day, I was wondering why I hadn't rung her myself. It was so clear that's what I should have done, but I wasn't thinking clearly, and simple decisions were out of my reach.

A couple of days later I received my fourth round of chemo and was half way through with treatment. I was unusually anxious because I'd never had Docetaxels and was concerned how my body would cope. As usual, I hated the first hour when they placed the Cold Cap on my head, but I had to keep reminding myself that it was worth it because although loads of hair had fallen out, it was thinning all over and not coming out in clumps. I could still get away with wearing a cute cap. It turned out in the end that I never had to wear my wigs, so the Cold Cap was definitely worth the agony.

During my fourth treatment Dr Simcock came into the Cold Cap room, shut the door and pulled up a stool in front of me. It was now just Peter, him and me, which alerted me I was about to hear something he didn't want anybody else to. He was right. I didn't even want to hear it, let alone other patients and staff members. He told me he couldn't be the support I needed because it might compromise his ability to treat me objectively. No doubt this speech was a follow on from the email I had sent a few days before.

I held his eyes with mine trying to tell him how much I was suffering inside. I felt like he understood because he seemed to be looking into my eyes, not just at them. He had told me in a very nice way that he couldn't be 'doing emotions' in this game, and I felt like an abandoned puppy with droopy watery eyes wagging my tail, hoping he'd change his mind and stroke me. He was speaking to me like a 12 year old and that was hard, however much I may have been behaving like one.

Trying to communicate my pain to him wasn't all a waste of time. After he had given me the speech, he gave me information on a place called The Bristol Cancer Healing Centre (now re-named the Penny Brohn Centre after it's co-founder). I believe my inner sorrow had a lot to do with why I had cancer again and why I may have had it 23 years ago, so this place appeared to be just what I needed to start my inner healing process. The timing couldn't have been better, as I had just read an article a couple of days before in a magazine dedicated to cancer, called ICON. It touched on treating the whole person – including the heart, soul, and mind. The Bristol Cancer Healing Centre was the kind of place where I could go and do that in addition to getting a quiet break from day to day responsibilities.

I knew things had to change. My situation could not remain the same. I was a mere shadow of myself, introverted and hidden away to the point I didn't even recognise myself anymore. Yes it was scary, but at least I had a chance. Not everything in my life was bad. I just had to get the balance right. I needed to figure out if this episode of cancer was helping in some way to come to terms with cancer so long ago, or was the cancer episode from so long ago making my journey through cancer this time so much more complicated? Everything was muddled in my mind. When I reacted to something, was it a ghost from the past coming to haunt me, or was I reacting to something from the present?

The following week, I observed that my diseased breast was now smaller than my healthy breast. It was a significant and important change. It meant that since receiving my first dose of Docetaxel, and learning about the Bristol Centre – a huge symbol of hope, the cancer inside my breast had reduced dramatically. It was working! Not only that, but my breast began to really ache, and I was assured this was a good sign. This hope went a long way and made me fight that much harder. I suddenly felt like I was winning, and subsequently started fighting for me, not just my family.

Chapter 43

Support

Having breast cancer and the subsequent treatment brought my life full circle with all my lifelong friends and family visiting, emailing, telephoning and sending gifts. I had gone years without speaking or being close to many of them and then suddenly there they all were: Alice, Wendy, Jill, Mom, Dad and my sister Tina and many others all showering me with love and affection. The amount of support I received was wonderful and pulled me through some of my darkest days. Yet I couldn't help worrying that all the fuss and attention would soon end and everything would go back to the same isolated world I lived in before. I realised I needed them in my life and was frightened of being alone again.

I considered the wonderful people who have made me who I am today, especially my sister Tina. Because she was the eldest of us three girls, she witnessed and replicated a lot of the dysfunctional behaviour our biological mother displayed. The worst mistake of all was abandoning her two eldest children. The pain she feels over that still threatens her sobriety to this day, but I keep reminding her that despite her mistakes in life, she's one of the most beautiful and soulful women I know as long as she isn't drinking.

In her darkest days, there isn't much Tina didn't experiment with sexually or drug wise. At one point she was even addicted to crack and heroine, but on her own she managed to detoxify and remains sober and drug free for over five years now. That's a huge a feat for somebody who has grown up without any parents or role models. She even went back to school and got a degree in hospitality and tourism. Despite all her faults, she has always tried to be there for me, and I am thankful for her weekly calls and daily emails throughout my treatment, as well as for her input into this book. She has gone through the pain of remembering with me so that we could bring together the pieces, and I know it's been excruciatingly painful for her too.

Email from Tina

I have been trying so hard to remember things from our childhood. I remember going to Kentucky Fried Chicken all the time. I can hear the leaves rumbling down the streets and feel the brisk air on my cheeks, and see the rosy colour in yours. There was the time when we lived in the nice mobile home, we used to play around in those old cars, mom dug up all kinds of old bottles and sold them on picnic tables. PK hitting the trailer with his car, mom grabbing us and running down the street hiding us in some bushes, watching PK drive up and down the street looking for her. I know I use to have nightmares in that trailer. Mom tore down one of the walls and made one big room for us girls, I don't know why. I think she did use some kind of drugs then. Remember the accident. We were all in snowsuits coming home from a party at Aunt Anita's house and just as we pulled into the driveway, a car hit us and we went into a great big oak tree in our driveway. Mom and Doug were really messed up. I know we stayed at Uncle Dicks and Cynthia's then. Remember when mom got that motorcycle? She was so funny, she got on it, and she hit the tank on the side of the trailer and broke the right blinker off. I remember some good times from then and a lot of bad like the pussy willow branches, and going to bed at daylight. I was always in trouble. I would try to do anything to please her and always failed. She hated me. I really felt that way. She cut my hair with such anger. I don't know if you remember when we were with that man, I guess she gave us to him, but I thought he kidnapped us, I still don't know. It really bothers me when I can't remember stuff. It is like an inner child is throwing a fit inside me. I wish I knew more about her. I have no sense of being close to anyone when I was younger, except you. I don't know of anyone whom I felt cared for by. I think that is so sad today. But there is no way of changing any of it and it sucks to start now, knowing how much I have missed out on, but I do realize it is better than never feeling that way. Someday I will get that in my head and really feel it. I love my son, but all I think about is losing him. Well not always, cause I am getting better about the feeling stuff. I just feel so alone sometimes, 'cause he wouldn't understand this stuff I am feeling. I love you and I need to go. Say hello to all.

Chapter 42

Meeting my inner voice

When I tried to book a weekend at the Bristol Centre they said they were fully booked. I felt really disappointed because I really thought it was meant to happen. Then I had a call informing me there had been a last minute cancellation for a five-day residential course. Originally Peter had said that a five-day course would be too long because there would be nobody to help with the children, but my mother was visiting and she was more than happy to look after them so I could attend.

I was excited to be going but also frightened beyond words. It meant travelling alone for four and a half hours at night to a destination I had never been to. It meant walking into the unknown, throwing myself into a group of people I had never met. This alone was causing me severe panic attacks. Because of my depression, I hadn't spoken to anybody other than my family and close friends for a very long time, and usually then it was only through email. I was scared I would say all the wrong things and be judged. Obviously my problems were so much worse than anybody else's, right? Despite my debilitating fear, I decided to do it anyway. This was going to be the beginning of my spiritual healing and road to recovery I had promised myself. I thought, *if I don't do it now, I never will.* Therefore, I packed my bags and headed into the unknown.

Journal entry upon arrival to the Bristol Centre

It's Sunday, 10th December 2006, and I'm now lying in bed of room B10 of the Bristol Centre. Elvis' Christmas songs are playing on the CD player, and I have two tea light candles burning (brought from home). It's very soothing and pleasant. Although, I am wondering why I've had to come so far away from my beautiful home to feel this way. The drive was hard. It was raining and the spray from the large vehicles in front made it scary at times. I have to say, it's nice to not be drinking this evening. My poor body needs a break. So, at least for the next 5 nights – it's tea total for me. I really hope this experience makes some life changes. I want to overcome my irrational fear of people. I want to be able to reach out to others and be a source of support. Show me how!

December 10th is the day James and I got married. It's hard to comprehend that it was 15 years ago when I made the first major mistake in my life (smile). Where does the time go? I hope I feel better tomorrow. I'm very panicky and nervy today. Like I could have a panic attack any moment. Peter left me a sweet note in my journal saying he loves me. I feel so sorry for him going through this with me. It must be so hard for him to watch me drink myself to death and hear my inner worries. He's beautiful to tolerate me the loving way he does. Going to fill in my questionnaire now.

PENNY BROHN CANCER CARE COURSE
QUESTIONNAIRE

1. How are you feeling? *Emotionally/Spiritually:*
Frightened, tired, bored! Anxious. I don't feel any

spirituality – just feel matter-of-fact, and a bit angry this is happening to me again. I find myself just not caring anymore – part of my depression. Empty inside.

Physically: Better than I am emotionally! Not too bad once I get over chemo. Very forgetful though and keep having panic attacks.

How stressful is your current lifestyle? I have a 7-½ month old, a two year old, a 3-½ year old, and a 12 year old, so I never get a break. I have no friends in the UK, so I lead a rather insular and isolated existence – which is stressful for me.

3. What major difficulties, upsets or stresses have you had over the last three/four years? Where do I start? I had two lots of back surgery whilst being pregnant, my 'biological' mother died (I was an older adoption), my little sister Kay died of cancer aged 21, I ran a <u>very</u> stressful business which I eventually closed down, I had three babies back-to-back – then I was told I have breast cancer!

4. What close and dependable support do you have now? *Personally:* My partner Peter. My American friends – we chat online.

From Health Care Professionals: Very limited contact with my oncologist.

5. Do you belong to a support group? If so, which one? No, but I wish I had enough courage to join one.

6. Do you have any complementary therapy, healing or counselling at present? No.

I filled out the questionnaire, but for some reason never gave it to them. Reading it now, even though I felt I was being very cautious with the true extent of my answers because I didn't want to appear a huge fruit-loop, it's very plain to see it's a wonder I didn't go BANG! sooner. There wasn't one aspect of my life that was truly happy or balanced.

It was humbling and a pleasure to meet the other 8 delegates, six of whom were terminally ill, and two spouses of somebody who was terminally ill. One woman had breast cancer for the third time, had had a double mastectomy and her hip replaced, but had never once been offered chemo or radiotherapy. She was always smiling and had a very warm aura to her. There was another older woman who had lung cancer but refused to have chemo. She kept nearly coughing her lungs up just like Kay did. Another woman had tumours all over her body, while a man around 50 had a rare blood disorder which was slowly killing him by shutting down all his major organs. Yet they all seemed to go on the best they could, not moaning in the least.

The first evening, I quietly lay in bed with candles burning full of inner stillness and peace. It was just what the doctor ordered – literally! With no pressures to perform, I felt so calm. A phone call home had told me all was fine, and despite my worry for my boys, I wasn't missing them too much. The following day I had a session booked with a psychotherapist that I was looking forward to and felt would be interesting. Then it was Art Therapy, an appointment with a holistic doctor and of course lots more meditation and relaxation sessions.

First thing the following day, I had my appointment with the psychotherapist. She used the usual counselling techniques I am familiar with, but did help me get to the nub of my main problem. Now that I recognise it, it seems as plain as day. She explained to me that as a young girl I had learned to live without a lot both physically and emotionally. Rejection was common and I always felt it was something I did, that I wasn't good enough and that's why people didn't love or nurture me. She told me I needed to learn how to take care of the young, fragile 7-year-old abandoned girl inside, and in order to do that, I needed to make time for myself. She asked me if I had a 7-year-old daughter, how would I look after her? I said I would do her hair, take her places, encourage her interests, and show her love and warmth by being gentle and patient. She asked me why I don't do things like that for myself. She was right. How could I have overlooked myself for so very long?

It was such a relief to be able to voice how it feels to be abandoned by your mother at a young age, and how it has affected consciously and unconsciously most choices I make as an adult. I expressed how the feelings of rejection made me feel lonely, unloved, and worthless. As I let the truth pour out of me, I suddenly saw how I was still carrying around the wounded and hurt feelings created by abandonment. I never felt good enough about myself as a person to look at myself through my own eyes instead of through other's because ultimately I thought, *how can I love me if my own mother didn't?* By recognising my emotional patterns and embracing the abandoned little girl, I was slowly empowering myself and learning how to love and care for me like I should have been taught by my mother.

In Art Therapy we had to throw together some kind of art that would express how we feel about living with cancer. I drew my glass teacup, which just happened to be sitting half full/empty in front of me. I felt it symbolised either the beginning of the end, or the beginning of the rest of my life. Would I fill it up and make cancer a positive experience, or would I watch what was left slowly evaporate away? I wanted to FILL it! I have a lot to give.

The comments back were insightful. Two women pointed out

how 'detailed and controlled' the picture was. They asked if being in control is an issue for me. I said, 'isn't it for all of us? Don't we all wish we had more control over cancer?'

The art therapist asked if my glass was half full or half empty. I said, 'Right now it's half full, but I struggle to always see it like that.' He asked what positive things I could do to keep it half full. I said I want to make myself stronger so I can write a book and share my experiences. I want to be there for others. I still had that option, whereas my fellow delegates had to live with the fact that they were in the process of dying. It made me so incredibly sad to know these wonderful people were losing their battle against cancer, and they were all such beautiful people with families. Why is life so cruel? Why did they have to go through this?

The therapists kept asking me what I wanted out of this experience, and each time I said something different. I wanted to express myself. I wanted to bring all the facts together. I wanted to learn how to relax and rest. I wanted to reach out and not feel so frightened anymore. I wanted to LIVE!

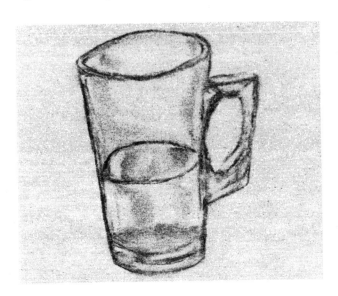

Following Art Therapy I had my appointment with a holistic doctor who told me which vitamins I should be taking, suggested a book and hypnotherapy to help with my phobias – namely, my irrational fear of people. He ended our session telling me he had very strong feelings I'd be OK, and as I left, he said, 'Remember, the glass is half full.'

The book he recommended was, *Wherever you go, there you are* by Jon Kabat-Zinn. The recommendation came as a result of me complaining about how disheartening it was to keep reading book after book that insinuated it was all my fault I had cancer, and if it wasn't that, it was extreme measures I should be taking to save myself. Weighed down by the 8 billion things I should be doing, I felt panicky, like a twitchy rabbit on the run. I had no inner peace. He said, 'Stop reading them then.'

Wow! What a simple idea; one that I hadn't even considered. He said, 'If they make you feel so unhappy, don't read them. Try reading this book…' and he wrote down the name for me. I went to the bookstore in the lobby of the Bristol Centre, bought the book, and started reading it straight away. It was to change the way I approach my life, my relationship with myself, how I connect with my environment, and how I handle stress. *Wherever you go, there you are,* is a book about mindfulness and meditation in everyday life and I would recommend it to anyone generally, whether they have had cancer or not. In reading it, I am reminded that I know the answers and they are inside me – not in books that claim they know how to save my life in ten easy steps.

The next day we were paired off with another delegate and told that one of us should ask the question, 'What makes you hurt?' and the other should answer. We didn't comment on each other's response – we only mentally took note and then asked the question again. When it was my turn to answer, the first thing that came to mind was how incredibly sad it made me feel that all the beautiful people in our group, myself included, were facing what we were. Then, of course, I mentioned my children and Peter. I was hurting that I might not be there for them in the future, and that I was hurting Peter by having cancer. Another thing I mentioned was how much my kidneys were aching from the last chemotherapy session. I was finding it difficult to meditate or relax with the waves of cramping.

On my last evening at the Bristol Centre I experienced very mixed emotions. On the one hand, I was missing my boys so very much. On the other, I wasn't looking forward to going home to a pot of stress. It had been so quiet and peaceful for me with no demands other than to look into myself for answers and truths. No screaming, no responsibilities, no expectations, no moaning, no cleaning, no cooking... I would miss the respite from all of that. The experience I had at the Bristol Centre made me aware of what I needed to change to be happier in life. I wanted to LIVE my life – not be a shadow in it. So many thoughts and emotions had passed through my heart and mind. I felt more me than I had in a very long time, and I was frightened of losing myself when I got home. In the beginning of my breast cancer journey, I told myself, 'Things must change' and now they had and I didn't want to go back.

Upon arriving home later that evening, I was not welcomed home by a hug or a kiss, or a 'how was it? I was not, in fact, welcomed at all. Peter came home later than usual, and upon his arrival home he avoided physical contact with me. When I asked why, he said something along the lines of, 'What did you expect? You go away for a week, and you expect me to be happy about it?' I felt like he had punched me hard in the stomach. I had been so positive and recharged until I came across him. Things were very bleak between us for some time after. I couldn't forgive him for not understanding.

Chapter 45

Looking for meaning

In an attempt to give meaning to my situation, I kept looking for reasons as to why I had cancer and ways to avoid it coming back. Was it my poor Western diet, my environment, the perfume I wore, my genes, bad luck, electric cables over my head, alcohol, red meat, bubble bath, microwave and satellite dishes, mobile phone masts, drinking out of plastic bottles or lack of expression? Should I move to the outbacks of Australia and bury my head in the sand just in case? The books I read on the subject revealed some interesting facts and statistics about a subject that makes no sense at all.

UK researcher Leslie Walker reported on a recent study that showed a staggering 17.5 per cent increase in survival 13 years after treatment in women who were taught relaxation techniques and, through hypnosis, to believe that their chemotherapy would cure them. The women who had achieved this huge rise in survival rate were those whom Walker called 'women who were too nice.' The medical description was 'women with a high level of social conformity' who tended to look after everyone else and bottle-up their own feelings. He also found an increase in immune function after relaxation and hypnotherapy. It goes on to say that another trick to learn is expressing your feelings in everyday life (not only in relation to diagnosis). Those who are too nice have suppressed immune function, so it's best to copy the Europeans and let rip with our feelings!

'Unacknowledged pain is subtly destroying many people's lives. We all know people who are out of touch with their pain – who have refused to let themselves feel their emotions. When we don't acknowledge our pain, it will be transferred into a bodily symptom, anger, or something equally destructive. We need to get rid of pain and anger before we can bring in love. When we hold negative feelings about our past, we carry these feelings to our present. Not only that, but we can make ourselves physically ill.' Susan Jeffers.

Another fact taken from *The Cancer Directory*, by Dr Rosy Daniel is 'Adrenaline exhaustion triggers a chain reaction causing the thyroid, in an attempt to compensate, to ultimately 'burn out.' The knock on effects on the immune and endocrine systems then leaves the door open for cancer to develop.'

There is a landmark study of more than 14,000 patients reported on in the New England Journal of Medicine that found survivors of childhood cancer have frequent and serious health problems. According to The Childhood Cancer Survivor Study, 80 percent of children with cancer become long-term survivors; however, the dark side to being cured is that by the time survivors are 30 years out from their cancer diagnosis, almost 75 percent of them have a chronic health problem and 42 percent die or have severe life-threatening conditions. The sobering statistics are that cancer survivors were 3.3 times as likely as their healthy siblings to have a chronic health condition, and 4.9 times as likely to have two or more chronic health conditions including second cancers, fertility problems, heart disease and kidney failure. At highest risk are children who had bone cancers (that would be me), brain tumours, and Hodgkin's lymphoma.

Most interesting was the book *Getting Well Again* by The Simontons who are worldwide leaders and pioneers in mind-body medicine. Their total approach to fighting cancer combines traditional medical management with psychological treatment to create the most favourable environment both internally and externally for recovery. Simontons' patients have a survival rate twice the national norm, and in many cases have experienced dramatic remissions or total cures.

Their book argues that the connection between cancer and emotional states has been observed for nearly 2000 years. Yet as the emerging sciences of psychology and psychiatry developed, traditional medicine lost interest in the problem. The result has been two very distinct bodies of literature and research, both disciplines working on the same problem often having little exchange of information. Therefore, they feel it is the separation of cancer from emotional states that is the new and strange idea.

I was particularly fascinated by the Chapter four that delves into the link between stress and illness offering many examples dating back as early as the mid 1800's demonstrating how emotions can cause illness.

Dr Thomas H. Holmes and his associates at the University of Washington School of Medicine undertook the task of validating these observations. They developed a scale that assigned numerical values to stressful events. Totalling the numerical values of all the stressful events in a person's life could indicate the amount of stress he or she was enduring.

The scale includes events that we all recognise as stressful, such as death of a spouse, divorce, loss of a job, and other painful experiences. Interestingly, it also includes events such as marriage, pregnancy, or outstanding personal achievement. Although they are positive experiences, they also demand a great deal of introspection and can cause unresolved emotional conflicts to surface.

Using the scale, Holmes and his associates were able to predict illness with a high level of statistical accuracy. Forty-nine percent of the people who had accumulated scores of 300 + points within twelve months on the scale reported illness during the period of the study, while only 9 percent of those with scores below 200 reported illness during the same period. Another twelve month study indicated that people with total point scores in the top third of those who participated in the study reported 90 percent more illness than did people in the bottom third.

Out of interest, I tallied my score. It didn't surprise me to find it was 496 based on my circumstances around the time I was diagnosed with breast cancer.

I've concluded that leading a healthy life is about balance. Furthermore, I believe there must be a connection between both our inner and outer environments. Honestly, if everything causes cancer to some varying degree, then why aren't all of us walking around with bodies full of tumours? We should educate ourselves about our internal and external worlds, bringing them both into focus. So much of our time today is spent in a gym working on our outward appearance, but how many of us spend time nurturing our spiritual being to make sure it is just as healthy?

I know we all suffer stress, but the connecting factor in people with cancer is how we handle that stress and how well we adapt to change. Two to three years ago, I didn't have any means of expression or interests of my own. I had forgotten how much I love to read, write, listen to music, sing, take photographs, and walk. When diagnosed, it didn't even occur to me to fight for me as well as my family. It was all about them. Today I'm trying to make time for me. It is difficult with four young boys, but when I can, I do.

Chapter 46

Finishing treatment

Nine days after I returned home from the Bristol Centre, I was back in hospital having my next to last treatment. This time Mom took me, and Peter's mother stayed with our boys while Peter went to work. It was a very different experience than the previous treatments. Mom and I sat in the large communal room instead of the usual stuffy Cold Cap room. I had been in the communal room before for various reasons, and although it was packed full of patients, I could have heard a pin drop. Nobody spoke to one another, and everybody's faces were drawn and pale. That day, however, Mom was there and she likes to talk.

I became very tired after receiving my chemo cocktail, so I stopped playing cards with Mom and shut my eyes to rest. I kept dozing in and out and each time I came to, I would hear Mom chatting with other patients. They were laughing and sharing thoughts about cancer and treatment. I eventually came around and joined in. I was doing it! I was reaching out and talking and nobody was judging me. I was so grateful to Mom for helping me break down some of my walls.

I only had one more chemo to go and then it was surgery. So deeply inspired by my fellow delegates at the Bristol Centre, I felt much better about the idea of a mastectomy after I returned home. It seemed a bit spoilt to moan. A boob is just fat anyways. It can be replaced. After all, I was in a secure relationship with a man who would always love me regardless. Moreover, even if I weren't, I'd never want to be with a man who put my boobs above me in our relationship. The upcoming radiation every day for 5 weeks was now worrying me most. My reasoning, as it turns out, is what is termed, 'minimisation.' I was trying to make light of the situation telling myself that there are others worse off and that I shouldn't complain.

What I really thought was neatly masked by a web of delusion. I would look at myself naked in the mirror and wish there was a way of saving my breast. I'd always liked myself in that department; they weren't perfect but they weren't bad either. I saw my breasts as defining my nurturing, feminine side. They're where my sons liked to rest their heads when they were tired, snugly or not feeling well and they were a physical pleasure for my lover too. I couldn't comprehend how losing such a symbolic piece of anatomy would affect my self-confidence and how others would feel about me. It was killing me; I didn't want anybody (including my doctors) to see me without my breast. My body would be covered in scars and I wouldn't be beautiful anymore. Giving myself a pep talk, I told myself at least I would still be here – a little worse for wear, but here none the less, and so it had to be.

The day had come and gone for my last chemo, and I felt like a heap of steaming manure. I had come crashing down from steroids and was depleted. Struggling to think straight, I wrote:

'Thank God I don't have to go through this again anytime soon. I'm even struggling to hold my pen. My hand aches and is shaking from weakness. That's it; I can now look forward to slowly recovering and building up

my immunity. Then I'm hoping sanity and emotional healing will follow. A friend and fellow cancer survivor from the Bristol Centre got in touch with me forwarding some photos of the group of us before leaving the Centre. She asked me if I was keeping up the positivity that I developed during our time there.

Have I – Fuck! Stooped over the table in floods of tears last night until 4 AM. I have so much pent up emotion and unexpectedly it all bubbles to the surface and all I can feel is doom and gloom. I haven't joined a support group, and I'm not sure when that is going to happen with four children to consider. My next step is surgery, and that brings to mind floods of emotions. I am frightened of surgery and recovery itself. I am frightened how I am going to feel about myself after my breast is removed. I am struggling to make up my mind about whether I want implants or reconstruction, and I don't know what is going to be the deciding factor. One moment I think, 'Yeah, definitely implants – BIG ONES TOO!' Then the next moment, I think it's not like me to have something as unnatural as that in my body. Then I think, 'but reconstruction is such major surgery and I'm frightened of surgery.' So, I really don't know...

Pumped full of steroids, I had pushed myself far too hard the day after my final treatment, going to Uckfield then Crowborough with the children in tow. Then I came home and made dinner and did two lots of laundry. It was no wonder I was in a heap crying my eyes out at 4 o'clock in the morning. Why do I always push myself so hard? Why do I always feel so guilty if I'm not being Super Woman? More importantly, why did Peter allow and expect me to be?

Two days following my last treatment, it was a bright sunny day, but the light hurt my eyes and my head throbbed. Peter and his mother had taken the boys out for a walk. Too weak and exhausted to contemplate fresh air, I stayed in. I'd had a hot bath and put on some snugly pyjamas and was going to rest. I pulled the curtains to in my bedroom and curled up in a foetal position on my bed thinking about how horrible I felt. I was in a state of complete emotional quagmire. Insecurity, sadness, vulnerability, anger, fatigue of spirit, and confusion all churned inside me.

I was too isolated in my own home with only children to talk to. I still had no friends in this country, and my conversations with Peter began lacking. With old friends and family from afar re-appearing in my life, I was finally feeling like I used to before I came to live in England. I felt a renewed sense of fight, and it really depressed me to think once I was cured that everything would go back to the way it was. Therefore, I wasn't going to keep pretending everything was jolly. It wasn't. The sooner I admitted that, the sooner I could try to change and make it better. I just wished I had a magic wand.

The more I grew and learned from my experience, the greater the divide between Peter and me became. Now not only was I frightened of moving forward generally, I was also fearful of losing my relationship. I was focussing on reaching out, learning, loving, and giving meaning to my life while he was thinking of our family unit. I struggled with the feeling of it not being good enough to hide away anymore, frightened of my own shadow and voice. I may die, and I didn't want to do it with huge regret hanging over me. I started to see that when I was concerned with something bigger than me, my fears greatly reduced. Peter just wanted to be the happy insular family we had always been.

Chapter 47

Surgery

Journal entry
Well, today is the day. I leave very shortly for the Nuffield Hospital in to have my left breast removed. Feeling very numb and my tummy is cramping. Took a Lorazapam last night that helped me sleep. Have to go now. The next time I write I'll be a woman with only one breast. Time to see what I'm really made of...'

Much later that day
'I am now flat as a pancake on my left side, which makes my right side look ridiculous on its own. My left arm is numb under my armpit until my elbow. I have two drains sewn in just under where they removed my breast – this hurts more than the main incision. I'm feeling better emotionally than I ever dreamed I would. I showed Peter my bandaged site, the bit I was dreading most, and his calm reaction put me at ease. He handed me a mirror and said, 'See, still the same person.' Bless him. I'm actually feeling a sense of relief right now. The cancer is gone. No longer part of my body. Now maybe I can breathe deeply again.'

Mr Zammit popped into my room at the end of the day to see how I was coping. He reassured me that he was happy with everything he could see during surgery. He did say, however, that the nodeS (plural) responded well to chemo – that there were residual cells left over from the cancer as proof they had been affected. Not great news when you consider that the more nodes affected, the less likely I will ultimately survive. So, now I knew it was plural and awaited confirmation on exactly how many.

It was very early the following morning, and I hadn't even opened my eyes yet, but I knew it was Mr Zammit coming through my door because he was always so cheerful and chatty with the nurses. I asked him to take a photograph with me, which he happily obliged. The difference in the way Mr Zammit and Dr Simcock relate to me is interesting. Mr Zammit is very personable and constantly reassures me through a small touch to the arm or hand. Dr Simcock rarely shares anything personal unless I drag it out of him, and very rarely touches me unless it's to physically examine me. Must be an Oncologist thing – keeping to and protecting himself just in case.

During Mr Zammit's visit, he suddenly jumped up and went to my garbage bin. He removed the plastic water bottles on top and found what he wanted to ask me about – the wine bottle. Not only did he find one, but two. I guess I must have stunk of alcohol, because he seemed quite sure he would find what he was looking for. I felt if I explained that Peter had helped me drink them that it may sound like I was making excuses so I just sat there feeling ashamed of myself. He told me it was 'OK;' he understood it was a hard time.

During my stay in hospital, I often came down from my room to sit outside on the patio facing the sea. It was where I liked to sit each time I came for a doctor's visit. My room was just above – best room in the house, I imagined. The days were gorgeous. The sun was so warm, and the view was spectacular. As for having had my breast removed, I wasn't sure how I felt yet. Right then it was OK, but I wondered if I was experiencing a delayed reaction.

I hadn't actually seen myself without the bandages. Perhaps that would shock me. It was obviously strange already, but the bandages seemed to hide the reality of it. My armpit really itched and felt swollen. I looked like a boy through my t-shirt. I had to carry around a pillowcase to hold my drains, which coupled with my bedclothes and my washed out face, made me look like a vagrant. I asked myself why I was feeling so weepy. I knew I was missing my boys who hardly recognised me anymore. What was really happening though was reality tapping lightly on my door.

During a visit with Mom and my boys, I showed Mom my... what should I call it now? It was certainly no longer a breast. OK, my 'surgery site,' and I could see she was deeply upset for me. I also showed Jiggy because he wanted to see my 'owie'. He looked very concerned that one breast seemed to be missing. He kept looking back and forth saying, 'One booby, and one owie.'

Tink continually wrapped his arms around my legs and said, 'I love you so much Mum,' and you know what? That made everything worthwhile. Who cared about boobs if it meant I got another day with my boys? Their smiles were the light of my life, and when I see myself in them, I glow with pride.

Later that evening, Peter came for a visit and we drank some wine and chatted for a while. Having been up with Laurence in the night and then at work until late, he was very tired. After he left, now alone in my hospital room, I decided I wanted to see what I'd become. I went into the loo, stood in front of the mirror, and began to remove my button-up pyjama top. I fixed my eyes firmly on a spot in the mirror careful not to look in the area of my missing breast as I slowly removed my top and then my bandages.

I stood topless not staring at my one breast, nor my one 'owie', but rather into my eyes. I saw how terribly tired, fragile, and frightened I looked.

I cautiously lowered my eyes to the area I had just uncovered. I saw it and then looked back into my eyes. What had I become throughout the years? How could I possibly be the same girl who wrote, 'See the birds. See the bees. See the butterflies fly around me?' I hardly recognised my own eyes anymore. Whom was this worn out woman staring back at me?

I began crying not for my lost breast, but for all the loss and pain that had made the courageous and brave woman standing before me – the woman that would give almost anything for a moment's rest. I felt my heart was so much closer to the surface now leaving it that much more vulnerable and exposed. Once again, being my own parent I took a tissue and dried my eyes. I thought to myself, *I am a fighter and stronger than I ever knew; I am not beaten. It's not my breast I will miss most – it is my innocence.*

The following morning Pam told me it usually takes 5 to 7 days before it hits home for a woman that they've lost their breast. I was a little ahead of the game. Apparently my numb response up until that point was quite normal, as was the fact that I was grieving now.

Another evening when Peter came for a visit, we were trying to guess what kind of cars Dr Simcock and Mr Zammit drive judging from their personality and ego levels. Peter said Dr 'Richcock,' as he calls him, probably drives a Porsche, and I said something a bit more humble like a BMW. Peter and I both agreed that Mr Zammit was a large silver Mercedes man. The next morning I asked Mr Zammit what they drive, explaining that Peter and I had a bet. It seemed we are both wrong. Dr Simcock's family only has one car – a people carrier, and he lets the wife drive it – apparently doing his bit for the environment. I wonder if it is more likely something to do with parking issues in Brighton. Mr Zammit drives a non-descript people carrier too. So there you go, not all doctors and surgeons are swanking around or swimming in it.

I felt disappointed that everybody involved in my care made a point of visiting me following surgery except Dr Simcock. He was at the hospital, all he had to do was pop up or outside and say hello, but NO! I decided he was fired. Even his secretary, who I had become quite friendly with, bought me a plant, some daffodils and fruit. As if that wasn't enough, she sat outside with me, Peter's mother and eldest sister, Mom and my boys for 45 minutes. She had even posted me a card. Pam came in on her day off to fit me with a 'comfy' (a temporary prosthesis), and Mr Zammit was in first thing in the mornings and last thing in the evenings. He and I even talked about Dragons Den and cars. I couldn't understand why Dr Simcock didn't take the time. It seemed cruel because he was the doctor I saw most during my treatment. I started to spiral down in my mind all the reasons ranging from, *oh my God, he must know the results of my surgery and is avoiding me!*, to *I knew it, he hates me!*

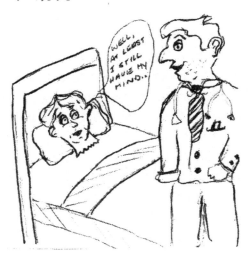

Six days after surgery I was finally home. Still feeling very tired and weak, I spent most of the first day in bed. My surgery site was very sore and itchy, but because the skin was numb, I couldn't scratch. I had a meeting planned with Mr Zammit the following week where he would fill me in on exactly how many nodes had been affected by cancer. Meanwhile, I was trying to get on my children's good side again. Laurence, the baby, preferred to go to Mom now, Jiggy was clingy and whiny and Tink wouldn't stop saying how much he missed me and what a 'lovely mum' I am. It broke my heart. On top of all of my worries, it was also Kay's birthday the next day. She would have been 25. It scared me to think of going through what she did; total hell on earth. Such a brave girl. I don't ever want to be that brave.

BLOG – 'Pathology Report'

Just found out yesterday the results of my pathology report following surgery, and guess what? Chemo kicked Cancer's butt! There was the odd cancer cell here or there, but generally, all that was left in my breast and nodes was the slimy trail left behind by the cancer after it crawled away and died.

I went in assuming it'd be bad news again – I'm getting used to hearing bad news lately. So! Imagine my surprise when my surgeon said there's a chance I may not even need radiotherapy after all. I told Peter I felt like doing something in wild abandonment to celebrate. He joked, 'You could always drop everything, run up to London, get drunk, strip off your clothes and make love under a fountain!' Hmmm... tempting; something I would have considered maybe 15 years ago. Instead, we settled on a whole-wheat ham sandwich with salad at Mrs Bumbles on the very cold and foggy sea front at Hove.

I sat there chewing on a few things – one being my

sandwich. I can't believe it's the end of my cancer journey. I feel like my life has been handed back to me. I want to grab it and run just in case somebody changes their mind. I thought of the things I've learned from my cancer experience; the wonderful new words I've added to my vocabulary – like Zoladex, Docetaxel, histology, oncotype, gene signatures, smart scalpel, transference, ruminating and a load of other really useful words that I'm positive will come in handy in the future. I also learned from my Oncologist that using the vernacular 'mouthy' in apologising for my behaviour means I've been in the UK too long!

I learned a few other useful things – like it takes a very special person to become an Oncologist; a job most sane people would pass up. Not that my Oncologist is insane or anything, and Surgeons aren't all bad guys waiting to cut you open or cut something off. Indeed, mine was very apologetic. I can't believe I'm about to say this, but I actually like him. After all, what would many others and I do without heroes like them?

Yeah, my journey has taught me a lot of useful stuff. Mainly, it's reminded me how precious my life is, how much I love my boys –big and small – and how much I want to give something back... Watch this space! So, time to put the cork back in the bottle and concentrate on staying cancer free and healthy. Whew! What a ride...

Following my good news from Mr Zammit, the bad news came that yes, I needed five weeks of radiotherapy, and Dr Simcock confirmed that because it was 4 nodes involved instead of 3, I jumped into the next category statistically in terms of survival. I didn't know how to feel anymore. One moment it was elation, and the next I was digging for a bone – something – God, please let there be some reason for all this pain. Then I thought, *I've been in pain most of my life. We probably all have.* I am not special in that way; life isn't easy. I just prayed that there was more to life than pain; there had to be more out there. I needed to know I wasn't going through all the discomfort of change and emotional growth to remain completely isolated and alone.

My scar was healing nicely, although it was very tight and I experienced 'cording' (pulling of the muscle that runs down the arm pit on the inside arm to the palm of a hand). The skin was also very sensitive to touch as if burned making it painful to sleep on that side. As for flexibility, I was doing well in that department. It helped having a 'Lumpy' baby who needed picking up all the time. I could nearly raise my arm all the way up above my head, but couldn't straighten it like my other arm. There were no problems with lymphatic swelling. I used 'scar gel' that Mom gave me from the States, also Palmer's Organic Olive Oil Butter with added with Vitamin E, and the redness of my scar was minimal. It looked very neat and clean.

As far as my other vanity issues, my eyebrows were finally starting to grow back — thank goodness. I looked like Ziggy Stardust without them. If only they could create a Cold Cap for eyebrows. My pubic hairs and eyelashes were also beginning to reappear. It was nearly three months before the hair on my head really started to grow. Before that it looked how I imagined a drowned rat would look. I had long, stringy pieces of hair that hadn't fallen out, and tufts of new growth under making it all look rather messy. However, as my son PJ said, 'At least you're here.'

AMEN.

As for my new self-image, I was trying not to think about it too much because I knew I wouldn't always look half boy on one side and half woman on the other. I had my moments though when something would surprise me like going to touch my breast because my phantom nipple ached and realising it was gone, or catching myself in the mirror whilst changing and I'd have a good cry.

Mom said seeing me with only one breast was like looking at me when I was 12 again. Breast or no breast, I still felt attractive — probably even more so than I looked. I didn't place my value in the breast I had lost. In fact, before my mastectomy I wondered how I was going to cope with anybody seeing me without a breast. As it happened, I didn't really feel less of a woman in the least. I knew I wanted to have surgery to replace what was taken, but I also felt the replacement would probably be better than the original. Moreover, who really cared about a flabby old sagging breast anyway? Believing this and putting my situation into perspective made coping a little easier.

'Honey, do you know where my boob is?' are words I never thought I'd hear myself say, but heard myself say regularly. I did find it quite humorous when I had to search the house for my breast wondering where I left it the previous night; another thing I never thought I'd have to do. Once I even found it in our airing cupboard because Tink had been playing with it and hidden it there. Sometimes I just had to laugh. It was a serious subject, but it didn't mean I couldn't find the humour in it too.

I think of some of the steps in my journey; the pain, the Bristol Centre, Peter, children, Dr Simcock, Mr Zammit, buying a Mini and driving around like a teenager again. It was so difficult and serious, but in retrospect, when wearing rose tinted glasses, there were aspects that were humorous too. When I had my one-on-one psychotherapy session at the Bristol Centre, I explained how I ended up there — that I had a wonderful, intuitive Oncologist who communicated a certain amount of understanding, which made me feel able to open up to him. I said, 'And when I did finally let out how I was really feeling, he ran 10 spaces back and gave me your number.' Even though I made it clear his reaction upset me, the psychotherapist couldn't stop laughing. I repeated to her again the bit about being upset, but she still laughed and before long I was laughing too.

Then I bought a 'Hot Orange' Mini convertible on a whim. To think what I must look like at my age, especially with my sons being wind blasted in the back. I laughed inwardly, possibly even outwardly, as I drove the Mini to Lewes one day to grocery shop. I looked in the rear view mirror to check on Tink, and realised what posers we must look like; both wearing our cool shades, hair flapping in the wind, ear to ear grins whilst listening to Cold Play and Van Morrison at top volume. The black veil was beginning to lift and I was beginning to feel it was safe to risk a smile.

BLOG – 'Oh What a Glorious Day!': *For those of you in the UK, I don't have to go into detail, but for my American pals, today in England was heaven – simple as that. When the weather here is good, there's no better place in the world, I swear to it. Since I share with you all of my 'dips', thought I'd also share with you a very profound and touching 'moment' I had earlier today.*

This afternoon in 80-degree warmth, I drove along in my Mini with the top down — of course, goes without saying — with my son PJ sitting next to me. I suddenly felt so incredibly moved and HAPPY! The wind was whizzing through my hair, the sun shining on my face, the lovely sound of David Sanbourn making love to his sax setting the scene. Warmth enveloped me. A feeling of 'FREEDOM AT LAST!' consumed me. Deep breaths in and out, lovely spring smells filling my tummy with a tickly feeling – the kind that makes you want to kick your legs like a two year old in an act of wee joy.

'I have hair! And the wind is messing it all up – YAY!' was only just one of my thoughts. More than anything, I was just there, not worrying, not anything. Just pure happy energy, in the moment… LIVING. Right here, right now. No tomorrow, no past; just me loving every second. Loving being me; loving me as a person and feeling good about me as a person – not a mom, not a partner. Driving along with my top down, the radio on, wearing my Kylie 'hot pants' shorts and tank top feeling like a sexy little minx! It's something that I haven't felt in a very long time. I nearly wept but didn't want to worry my son.

I've been down for so long that I had almost forgotten what I was fighting for. For so long it's been about surviving for others. I always put others first – ALWAYS. So, to have a 'me' moment was a blessing. It's renewed me. I can feel the old Lora Lee starting to surface again – except a bit better this time! I feel I could explode with energy and optimism. Channelling all this energy is my next stretch. My next hurtle. One moment I was frightened to stop chemo, to leave the side of my Oncologist (Richard, my 'father-hen') in fear of the stepping back into the world.

Today prodded me to stop trying to cling and avoid…. just BE. Be at Peace. Be happy. Be mad. Be sad. Be whatever you feel like right then. Right there. Who knows what tomorrow will bring. Oh what a glorious day… MY DAY!

A week later and once again I felt like I was losing my mind. I was seriously and deeply confused. I had to do something, speak to a professional of some sort. I feared my relationship wasn't what it could or should be, and it was dividing me in two. We were so happy, or at least I thought we were, before my cancer diagnosis. Now I didn't feel connected to Peter anymore. I was scared. I asked myself, *Why did I have to get cancer again? I was finally sorting myself out, was where I always wanted to be – perfect handsome man, beautiful children, secure home, building a new home...* Then, like always in my life, the carpet was pulled out from under me and I felt sick and dizzy inside. I really wasn't thinking clearly anymore. I couldn't feel love for Peter and I didn't know why. I knew I did. I knew I should. I was full of life that wanted to explode, but I knew this would probably hurt me as it always did – so I remained in a spot that made me miserable, but at least I was safe and my children had a normal home.

I read in *Feel the fear and do it anyway*, 'When you choose to remain stuck simply because you don't want to upset your mate, you become resentful of the fact that you have not had your chance to grow. Ultimately, the relationship becomes very strained, and it is not unusual for its breakdown to occur anyway.'

Then I thought, *maybe I should just die. Then nobody could blame me for leaving them.* That wasn't a choice for me to make; I may die even if I didn't want to. Why God was I thinking like this? I desperately needed to feel like part of a bigger cause with a sense of purpose so I would stop feeling so alone. I felt like screaming at the top of my lungs. My coping mechanism throughout had been looking down the neck of a wine bottle, or more precisely, BOTTLES. Even that wasn't working anymore, and the person hurt by it most was me. I really needed to do something to help myself. Things as they were simply weren't good enough, and if I waited for Peter's permission to reach out, I'd be waiting a mighty long time. I decided I was going to start doing things for myself, and Peter would just have to catch up. I had to believe that despite him feeling threatened by all my changes, he really did want what was best for me and that he would ultimately love the positive changes in me.

In an effort to bridge the gap that had formed between Peter and me, I asked Peter one evening after I put the boys to bed, 'Hey, fancy working up an appetite before dinner?' I really felt like I needed sexual expression and intimacy. Peter said he needed another glass of wine first.

Usually we don't have to think about the steps of getting into bed, but this was the first time I didn't know what I should do. The lights were on and I questioned if I took off my bra, would seeing me without a breast kill the moment for Peter? I felt shocked at the thought. It hadn't been a problem to date. In fact, we usually had a laugh about it. For instance, when my prosthesis fell out into the roasting pan when I was bending over checking the potatoes. I couldn't stop laughing at the absurdity of it. I know others may feel a pang of sadness at the thought, but at that moment it just made me laugh. Not tonight. Tonight I was actually worried that the sight of me would revolt Peter. I decided to leave my bra on and climbed into bed next to Peter. As he began to kiss me and carefully avoid touching either of my breasts, I began to quietly cry and didn't stop until after we made love and he had left the room. I don't think he even noticed.

Chapter 48

One step at a time

The goal post kept changing as I advanced through my stages of treatment. One moment I was saying, 'I'm really just worried about chemo', then it was 'I'm really just worried about surgery' and now it was radiotherapy. There's a lot of truth in the saying, *one step at a time.* If I had focussed on every aspect of the treatment laid out before me, I couldn't have coped. Instead, I tried to take it in bite-size pieces and just concentrate on what I needed to overcome now – not months down the line. When I did think too long and hard about the road ahead, I went into a depression and wanted to give up. Indeed, if we all knew what would happen months down the line, would we be tempted to give up and miss part of our journey? As it turned out, I loved my appointments to RT (radiotherapy). It meant I was able to drive my Mini with the top down in gorgeous sunshine, listening to music and feeling peaceful for at least an hour a day.

I woke up on my own in PJ's room one night not long after surgery. I had moved in there as PJ was gone at his dad's and Peter was keeping me awake with his snoring. I had settled into a deep comfortable sleep when suddenly my eyes popped open and I was wide-awake. The first thought that came to mind was,

I really love being me! Then the sadness followed because I remembered I had breast cancer and what that may mean. The highs and lows I have gone through in my breast cancer experience have been either heaven or hell. Sometimes, unbelievably, I am thankful it has changed me for the better and made my life so much more full. Then at low points, I think to myself, *what good is a mind if it's going CRAZY?* And yes, there were many times when I questioned my own sanity.

In between surgery and starting radiotherapy, I had a lot of time to think. I decided when my treatment was finished I wanted to celebrate life and living in the moment, so I invited my life long friends Alice and Jill to come to Paris with me – my gift to all of us. I was still worrying about feeling lonely and isolated once treatment finished, so it was something very positive to look forward to.

After organising my trip, I spent time looking back on some of the things I had written. I could see so many things I couldn't see at the time. I suppose much of it was down to feeling as if I was no longer the rat running around in the maze trying to find the cheese. I was now seeing the larger picture. Sometimes I liked what I saw, and other times I felt embarrassed I could be so naive. I enjoyed that Peter and I were still together – strong and proud – after so much time and tribulation. It was a soul destroying time for both of us, but we both wanted it to work, and were willing to do what it took to be together in the end. In fact, I've recently begun to realise how fulfilling a long history with somebody you love and who loves you in return can be. There's something heartening about sharing comforts and security, particularly during hugely insecure and trying times like these. I began to consider that maybe things weren't as bad as I thought.

One evening, Peter's sister came around and as we ate the

scrumptious dinner she had cooked for us, we spoke of our experiences of breast cancer. The more I read and speak to other people about their journey, the more I realise how so much of what I have gone through is typical stuff. If only I knew that at the time, maybe it would have been easier to get through.

Chapter 49

Radiotherapy

Radiotherapy was a breeze compared to my chemo treatment and surgery. The only gripes I had were when a machine was down and I forced to wait up to two hours for my ten-minute session, or when I had to queue for an hour for a parking space. Luckily that didn't happen often. When I was forced to wait, I met some incredible people and I was reminded how indiscriminate cancer is. I met a reputable architect, a lorry driver, a managing director, a couple of house wives, a model, some young and some old.

In my set-up session, a radiologist took my photograph to ensure no confusion about who they were meant to be treating in the future. Then they asked me to remove my top. We were in a large, cold room and it felt awkward to just remove my top, especially considering I still had one breast I could remain modest about, so I asked the two radiographers if they had a gown. They looked at me as if I had asked for a glass of champagne. One immediately replied, 'no' very flatly, no excuses made. The other radiographer said, 'Actually, we do have these new tops we haven't even used yet' and he went to fetch one. What he came back with was great. It buttoned up the front and also buttoned at the shoulders so that either side could be let down for treatment. I used it for the duration of my appointments and was very thankful that I didn't have to bare all each visit. It was small things like that which made me feel more human again, not just another case.

The treatment itself only took a minute or two; it was the positioning and aligning that took the remaining nine or so minutes. I had to lie on a cold metal bed and put my arm up over my head into a device to hold my arm absolutely still. The radiographer aligned the laser from the machine above precisely to the tattoos they had marked on my surgery site. They twisted and poked me until I was exactly where I needed to be and then left the room. A loud buzzer resonated throughout the large darkened room indicating radiation was in progress. If it weren't for the noise, and the subsequent darkening of skin over time, I would have questioned if they were actually doing anything at all.

There was a nice chap, Simon, who was chatty. He and a couple of the younger girls made the daily appointments a bit more fun. I also really liked the parking attendant. He knew the scoop on everything happening within the cancer centre. You wanted the latest gossip – he was your man!

Half way through my RT sessions, I asked Simon why they always asked me my name and date of birth – they obviously knew who I was by now. He said that besides being legally obliged, sometimes when a machine was broken down and there was a long wait, some patients would try to jump the queue by claiming they were somebody else when a name was called out – hoping that once they were in the treatment room, they wouldn't be sent away again. Anarchy in the RT Department! I kept playing this comical scene in my mind of the old guy in a wheelchair trying to sneak in unnoticed – the devious child still very much alive and kicking. I did feel very sorry for those who had to sit there for hours even though they were so weak they could hardly hold their head up. I suppose I felt for all of us.

With only a few more sessions left, I started thinking about the daunting prospect of getting on with life and rebuilding what had been torn apart. I wondered if Dr Simcock would shake my hand or send me a letter marking the end. I mean, what do you do at the end of treatment? It was all so strange to contemplate because cancer had become my life and soon everything would abruptly end.

Alice arrived and accompanied me the last day of my radiotherapy treatment before the three of us set off to Paris. It was a gorgeous summer's day so we were able to drive to Brighton with the top down. It was the first time I had seen her in thirteen years, and as luck may have it, a RT machine was broken down and there was over an hour's wait. I took her to a coffee bookstore and we sat, drank coffee and caught up on what had been happening in each other's lives. I felt so at ease – as I always had when we were young. We laughed about almost everything, exchanged stories, drank the rest of our coffee, and headed back to the hospital.

Two days later, we were in our hotel room in Paris. As Alice, Jill, and I got ready to go and see the Moulin Rouge, I took off my top and bra and showed them my surgery site. It was burnt and crispy from the 25 sessions of radiotherapy. Jill looked a little uncomfortable with it, showing signs of pity while Alice looked at me and said, 'God, that looks really good. It's a really neat scar – as a Tattoo Artist I've seen a lot worse.'

'Really? I feel like I look like a boy now.'

'A pretty HOT boy!'

Once again, Alice had a way of making everything seem better.

Chapter 50

Integration

Alice and Jill had come and gone. Paris had come and gone. Peter and I would begin normal life again – whatever that was now – free of hospital appointments, treatment, and cancer. I really didn't know what to do with myself at this point. Cancer had taken over my whole life, and now I was supposed to pretend it never happened and just move on. Not knowing what else to do, I decided it was time to implement some of the things I had promised myself at the Bristol Centre. I booked healing and counselling sessions to treat my emotional wounds.

Through a positive attitude, I began to find value from everything that has happened to me. Consequently, I started a visualisation program designed to attract positive energy. It goes back to how cancer starts in the body in the first place. A body constantly creates rogue cells genetically tweaked or flawed. They have no boundaries and disobey the rules, going around like naughty children doing whatever they feel like (a bit like my sisters and me when we were young). Usually our bodies, through our immune system, are able to recognise these gangsters and disarm them, but in the case of cancer, the gangsters wear a mask so our bodies don't recognise them as being bad guys. And as do many bad guys, they start gathering and loitering until the space they occupy is finally too small for so many big guys. Therefore, they travel and set up camp elsewhere and start the process all over again until a body is riddled with them and can no longer cope.

In my visualisation, I try thinking outside the box. I imagine the entire world is just one dot on someone's fingernail, and that I am a mere cell going about my own business and fulfilling my functions. For some reason, in my small life, the body around me keeps recognising me as a rogue cell. I imagine this is because of my bad, negative energy. The womb around me isn't getting what it needs, so now I too try masking myself as a positive force with a purpose to serve the body around me and to fulfil my role strongly and with clear intent. I will not allow other, stronger cells to bully me and take away my shine.

My counselling sessions were very helpful too. By the end of my first appointment I was sweating. I sat there and rattled away thinking, *God, this is me I'm talking about! I went through all of this and I talk about it as if I'm talking about the weather.* My counsellor told me I didn't have to talk about things if it bothered me too much, and I said, 'Oh no, I'm used to telling my story.' What I wasn't used to was connecting the story to me. It was as if I was talking about somebody else altogether.

I arrived at the healing centre for my fifth counselling session on a very warm summer's day. I tapped on the door with the large brass knocker and my counsellor opened the door and welcomed me with a warm smile. 'Hi Lora Lee. Come in.' I made my way into the lounge and sunk into the armchair. Every time I came into this room I felt a comforting energy envelope me. It was decorated in soothing creams and the walls were a turquoise blue. I breathed in deeply a couple of times trying to shed the stress I brought with me.

'So, how are you?' she asked.

'I'm OK' I said with a chirp and a smile as I always did. 'I've been so busy with my book, the boys, our new house, healing, and another project I've started. I haven't had any time to myself. There's never any let up. I really want to start a writing course, or maybe a photography course. It would be difficult with the children, but I'm sure I could manage. Isn't this weather lovely? I got to drive here with my top down. I love driving. Actually I feel pretty tired today. Did I mention the book I just read, *This Book Will Save Your Life*? It was quite humorous, but there was also an undercurrent of enlightenment. It was told tongue in cheek and took a poke at the Los Angeles over –the-top lifestyle. I really related to the central character and his emotional thawing out after years of being frozen and emotionally dead inside. The fact that it led him to a place exactly like the Bristol Centre, and the hilarious comparisons, makes my experience seem so absurd and I'm able to appreciate the funny side of that part of my journey. It was really good. You should read it. How are you?'

She didn't say anything. Instead, she let me sit in a pregnant silence. The longer I sat there not talking, the more I began to listen to what was going on inside. Up until this point I had been using the sound of my own voice to distract myself from feelings. Who was I trying to fool? I didn't come here to tell her how busy I was, or give her a book review. I couldn't do it any more, there was no place left to hide. I suddenly felt my pain leak down my cheeks. She handed me some tissues but didn't interrupt. It felt so good to embrace my fear and pain instead of running from it. When I stopped crying I said, 'Wow! Where'd that come from?' and for once true counselling began. Throughout our conversation, I started to listen to my heart when I said something, and questioned why I said it at all, realising it must have been of some significance. Slowly, slowly I began to scrape away at the surface of my sedimentary soul and discovered to my joy that I was a marsh mellow deep inside and it was time to come out and play.

The one thing that came out of my healing and counselling sessions was that I realised I didn't have to keep dying inside. I did have options. I could let go of resistance and let in the possibilities that my world has to offer. By saying 'no' as I had done up to this point, I was being a victim; I was blocking and fighting against opportunities for growth and challenge. By saying 'yes' to all aspects of my life, I was giving myself hope.

Chapter 51

Sir Lancelot

On another deliciously warm day in the beginning of August, I sat outside Sainsbury's in Haywards Heath waiting for an appointment with Dr Simcock. I had just come from a healing session where it took everything in me not to burst into tears over saying good-bye to him. I know he told me repeatedly that he was not abandoning me, that he was going to still see me every six months, but in my eyes it wasn't the same. Our doctor/patient relationship was vastly reducing and today was to be my final appointment for quite a while. I was feeling incredibly sad and shaky inside. I waited in my 'Mini Molly' car for over twenty minutes trying to compose myself before going into the hospital.

This was the meeting I had been looking forward to for over a year – the one where I got my handshake and pat on my back and am sent on my way, free of cancer and doctor's appointments. It was also the meeting I had been dreading. Frightened of being sent on my way, I longed for more doctor appointments to reassure me my cancer would not be coming back.

I checked in with reception and took a seat in the waiting area. I picked up a magazine, quickly thumbed through some pages before throwing it back onto the table. I adjusted my legs and feet several times, sat forward, sat back, and then sat forward again. I fiddled with the handle on my purse then rubbed my tummy to ease the cramping. Finally Dr Simcock called me into his office.

I was anxious and nervous as I took my seat in front of him. I hadn't seen him at the Ashdown Hospital before so it brought a new dynamic of unfamiliarity between us. He seemed a bit hyper and a little unfocussed as he started his, 'Well done – you've made it' speech... 'Here you are, a year down the line and through your treatment' he paused for effect. I gave him big eyes and raised happy eyebrows. 'It's been tough, but you handled treatment well...' A tilt of my head to the side, and stitched eyebrows communicated my sadness. 'And we feel very positive that the treatment has had a systemic effect and that you are now cancer free. As far as we can tell, you are cured.' Big smile and raised happy eyebrows again. 'So how have you been?'

Wow. That was it? I had been waiting for over a year for that speech? I had been climbing this mountain, slowly clawing my way up to the summit only to be met by this pathetic wave of anti-climax, and you know how much I hate that! Gosh, I didn't even get a handshake. Not even a pat on the back.

I was deep in concern over feeling left high and dry, whilst Dr Simcock leaned back in his chair. He crossed his arms and his stretched out legs creating a comfortable barrier between him and me.

'How's your nipple?'

I sat there dumbfounded and confused for what seemed like an eternity, but was in fact nana-seconds. I repeated with question in my tone and a raised inquisitive eyebrow, 'Nipple?'

He said, 'Nipple' as if it's a simple question – answer it.

I repeated the same comment with the same inflection and the same eyebrow, and he finally realised his mistake and smiled rather sheepishly. To ease the tension I said, 'I don't have a nipple. Remember?' with more raised eyebrows and half a smile in an attempt to say I was OK with his faux pas. Inside, however, I shrivelled inwardly that I had to draw attention to the fact that I had no left breast, and with deep hurt that he didn't remember one of the hardest things I've ever had to do. Suddenly Sir Lancelot appeared a normal man again.

His embarrassment embarrassed me, so I quickly diverted attention away from all the embarrassment by changing the subject to my leg that received radiotherapy 23 years ago. He happily complied, and tried to show me he did remember most things about my case by bringing them up at in-opportune moments.

At the end of the meeting we stood momentarily by the door making small talk. He then opened the door and I exited. As I walked into the hospital corridor, I turned around to say goodbye. He held his arm out and framed my face with his extended hand. 'Bye' he said briskly turning around and disappearing back into his office. That was it. I should have been feeling elated, but I didn't. I should have been feeling a sense of freedom, but I didn't. I was aching as I walked free of the hospital and cancer treatment. I felt similar to how I felt the day I walked out of the hospital with my first-born in my arms. I was thinking, *are you really going to let me walk away with this precious life? Do you really trust me enough?* And despite all my preparation for the next thought, it still persisted like a tic. 'Now what?'

It used to be OK to sit inside my four walls; it was safe and I was comfortable. I was also very alone. I didn't want to feel that way anymore, so I made having cancer a reason to be pulled out of my shell. It had been the most painful experience of my life. Having a person whom I trusted, whom I believed cared for me to guide me through and give me a reason to please and perform was crucial. Somebody who understood the process I was in, and felt my pain with me. Dr Simcock had become that person, and as I walked away from him, I felt heavy in my heart as I asked myself who would pay attention and praise me for all my hard work accomplished, for how far I'd come? With nobody to hold my hand, I took baby steps away from my 'father hen' into the real world, and it hurt with every heartbeat. Now I was exposed and still alone.

Chapter 52

Reaching out

On recommendation from Dr Simcock, I attended a two-day conference at the Hilton in Brighton being offered by the Breast Cancer Care Organisation. It was an opportunity to meet with a group of about 45 other younger ladies to discuss things that affected us during and after treatment.

On the first morning following breakfast and before the conference started, I went outside to get some fresh air. At 8:00 AM it was already about 75 degrees, and there wasn't a cloud in the sky. People were everywhere, but it was strangely quiet considering the numbers. It reminded me of San Francisco and I had a strong urge to go home, pack my bags and move back to California and live by the ocean.

I sat on a bench along the walk in front of the sea. Whilst looking out at the view in deep thought, a group of about 10 younger athletic men ran past me down to the sea. Without speaking, they all began to remove their tracksuit bottoms and t-shirts leaving Speedo style bathing shorts on. Could this view get any better? All the men plunged into the sea. Two larger, rounder men waited on the beach as the young men treaded water. I imagined music from Chariots of Fire playing, and thought the scene belonged in the movie Dead Poet's Society. Within ten minutes they were out, drying off and heading up the beach.

That was my queue to end my daydream and go back to the conference. Back inside I told some of the women what I had seen and they informed me that the men were members of a cricket team staying at the hotel. God I wish I were single sometimes. Not that they would want a 38 year old one breasted woman with four children and a chequered past.

That night a large group of us went down to the beachfront and sat outside Gemini's bar listening to a duo perform. It was so atmospheric. Some people were dancing and some were playing volleyball on some sand they've obviously imported from Dubai. It was the most charming, warm and perfect evening.

Chatting with the other women, we all agreed there are some real idiots who seem to always say and do the wrong things when speaking to us, the 'breast cancer survivor.' **Example No. 1:** 'Oh! You have breast cancer. My best friend's mum had breast cancer. She died.' **Example No. 2:** 'God, you are looking amazing.' We, the breast cancer survivor, are thinking, 'Oh dear! I must have really looked like shit before!' And finally, my personal favourite, you tell somebody you have or had breast cancer and the first thing they do is stare alternately at each breast with the question, 'Which one is it?' written all over their face. When I told Peter this happens, he said, 'I should go around telling women I have penis cancer!'

I remember saying to somebody at the very beginning of my breast cancer journey that I used to feel special beating cancer the first time around because it was so rare and now that I was facing such a common kind of cancer, I felt like just another statistic. As I sat with all the wonderful women at the conference, I realised for the first time how comforting it is to have a type of cancer that affects so many. I've joined one of the most supportive and warm-hearted groups there is, and I'm thankful to be a member.

During the conference in our discussions we learned there are seven 'Possible Stages of Transition' one can pass through in dealing with traumatic experiences in our lives. They are:

Step 1:   Shock and Immobilisation

Step 2:   Reaction

Step 3:   Minimisation ('It could be worse')

Step 4:   Self Doubt

Step 5:   Letting Go

Step 6:   Testing – Exploring new options and different ways of coping

Step 7:   Search for Meaning – A conscious striving to learn from the experience

Step 8:   Integration – New self-concepts and understanding

So, that's me finished with breast cancer then! I'm interested to know why there are eight steps to '7 Possible Stages?'

At the end of our final day, I found myself looking around at all the youthful faces I had come to know over the past 48 hours. They were watching and listening intently to the speaker, and it suddenly dawned on me that some of us wouldn't be here in five years time. It was hard to believe when we all looked so healthy and full of vitality. Who will it be? Which one of us will lose our battle and why?

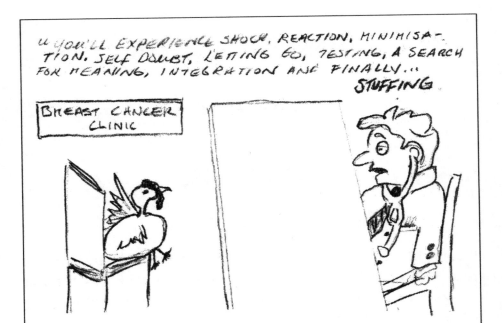

Chapter 53

Stuffing

I saw Mr Zammit to discuss the way forward with my reconstruction. Whilst he examined my scar he said, 'Yes, the scar is darker on either side…' I quickly cut him off explaining, 'That's because of radiotherapy. The beam hits either side of the scar first upon entry and absorbs a stronger ray.' I got a sweet smile that told me, *Yes, I know this already, but you're funny.* And of course I realised he did. I quickly added, 'Like I needed to tell you that!' The breast care nurse concurred with a laugh. He did say that my scar was healing beautifully (which he would do, of course, considering it is his handy work), and then commented that my skin was remarkably soft which is down to me looking after it.

We decided that in order to get my reconstruction over in one operation, and because the skin where my natural breast used to be was so tight, that I should have skin and muscle taken from my back and moved to the front in order to fit an implant. There wasn't even enough skin remaining for an inflatable implant without transfer of skin from somewhere else. I also opted to have an implant in my right breast to aid symmetry and my peace of mind in the future. Mr Zammit referred me onto another surgeon named John Boorman.

Having already met with Mr Boorman a few times, the day had finally arrived for my reconstruction 9 months and two days after losing my breast. If pushed, I could probably tell you the exact hours, minutes and seconds too. Following being checked into room 20 of the Mc Indoe Centre in East Grinstead, Mr Boorman came in dressed in his blue surgical attire and drew blue lines all over me where he was intending to cut. I tried not to think about how long the surgery would take or how much he was going to be cutting. Instead, I preoccupied my mind and time by posing for photographs of Mr Boorman doing his handy work on me.

After Mr Boorman left my room, an anaesthesiologist visited. I asked for a pre-med because I was literally shaking inside out. I have an irrational fear of being anaesthetised, worrying that I may never come back again. I am also extremely apprehensive of being completely out of control of my bodily functions. It didn't help that the anaesthesiologist just happens to live two houses down from where we are building our new home. Nice way to meet my new neighbour. I just hoped he wouldn't be in the room when they inserted the catheter into my bladder. As I juggled all my thoughts and fears, the anaesthesiologist struggled to find a vein (the portacath I had during chemo was taken out during my mastectomy). It took four or five attempts before they found a vein in my ankle. Once hooked up, it was only a matter of seconds before my lids struggled to stay open and I switched off like a light.

When I came to, my eyes were blurry from the gunk they had kept my eyes moist with during surgery. I believe the whole operation took five hours. My first vision was of Peter looking over me. Mr Boorman was in the room within moments checking his handy work. Because I would need to be checked every hour, they didn't bother with wrapping bandages over my wounds. They simply put a large pad over so I was able to see the results straight away. I complained that the left looked bigger than the right, and asked why the right breast looked such a different shape. Mr Boorman politely explained that it was early days and when things settled down, we would have a clearer idea of what adjustments, if any, need to be made.

The resident doctor accompanying Mr Boorman took offence to my immediate criticism asking me if I knew where I was. He went on to give me history of how The Queen Victoria Hospital adjacent to them was leading the way in surgical procedures since the war. The surgeons, who work for both establishments, were the finest I could ask for. It didn't stop me from continually questioning what was happening to my new breasts, though. Peter said as he walked passed the nurses station to leave, he overheard the same doctor griping to one of the nurses, 'What on earth did she expect for God's sake?'

I had three drains removing excess fluids from my wounds. This time, however, I brought with me a cute white bag to put the bottles in so I didn't look like a vagrant carrying around a pillowcase. The nurses loved it, asking me if I was off for a bit of shopping as I went for a walk down the corridor.

I was the only patient I saw walking around. I am accustomed to a fast pace life, so after two days of being in bed, I needed to move. I could only read so much in one day, and I don't watch much TV, so I was extremely bored. By the end of my fifth day, I was contemplating calling a taxi to pick me up and take me home. Luckily on the sixth day, Mr Boorman said the nurses could remove the drains and I could go.

Foolishly, in my usual style, I did far too much upon my arrival home. I was picking up Laurence, cooking, hoovering, and doing laundry. Mom and Peter begged me to stop, but I knew better. Within two days, my right breast was twice the size of the other and flaming red. I went back to see Mr Boorman and he put me on strong antibiotics and demanded I rest. I did the best I could. It was touch and go as to whether I'd be home for Christmas or back in room 20 of the Mc Indoe Centre.

My breasts showed slow signs of improvement and I managed to get through the holiday season. After New Years, I had another superficial infection along the scar on my right breast. Once again, he put me on antibiotics and again the infection cleared.

Since then everything has settled and when I wear a bra, you wouldn't even be able to tell I had surgery. The bra covers the line on my back and the scars up front, and the pertness of the implants looks so youthful – I wished I had opted for implants following the birth of my first son when everything started going south. I will have to go back to have a nipple reconstruction and some slight adjustments, but other than that I am now officially finished with treatment and surgery.

Chapter 54

Moving on

What is life now? It's getting back into a normal routine with my children and rebuilding my relationship with Peter. No more doctor appointments to take me away from their sides. It's building our new house up on the hill, making it a home together and appreciating the breathtaking views it commands. It's giving up the illusion that any one of us has any control over the future and what it may or may not bring. It's feeling part of a community and healing my inner self by giving something back. I have met new friends through my experience, and continue to employ the techniques I learned along my journey. My life now is just that – right here and now. No more dwelling on the past – what's done is done. I am looking forward to what today has to offer, and am thankful for the lessons of yesterday. If I can reach out and touch at least one person with my story, my life will be validated.

Why not come visit me on Myspace:

http://www.myspace.com/serendepityuk